R.

81

CATTLE BEHAVIOUR

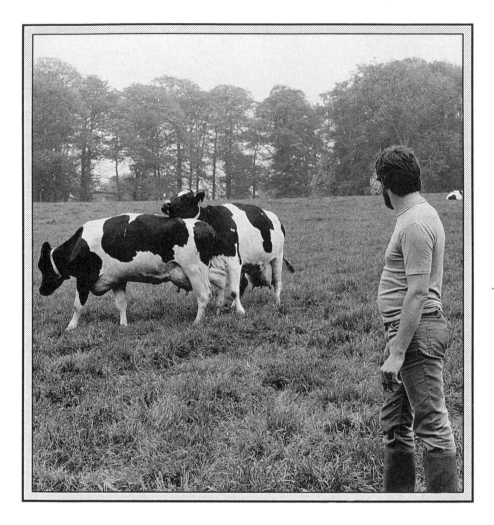

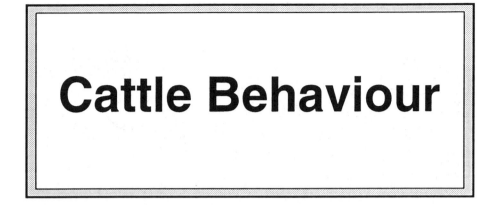

Cattle Behaviour

C. J. C. Phillips

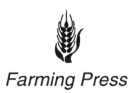

Farming Press

First published 1993

ISBN 0 85236 251 X

A catalogue record for this book is available
from the British Library

**Published by Farming Press Books
Wharfedale Road, Ipswich IP1 4LG,
United Kingdom**

Distributed in North America
by Diamond Farm Enterprises,
Box 537, Alexandria Bay, NY 13607, USA

Front cover photograph: Genus/David Platt
Back cover photographs: Nicholas Spurling;
Joe Everett/The Environmental Picture Library; Jeremy Williams

Cover design by Andrew Thistlethwaite
Phototypeset by Galleon Photosetting
Printed and bound in Great Britain by
Butler and Tanner Ltd, Frome and London

CONTENTS

A colour section precedes page 151

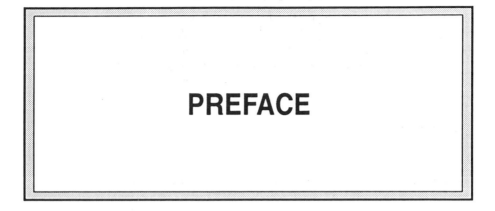

PREFACE

Studying the behaviour of cattle is one of the youngest and the oldest
sciences. The first students of cattle behaviour were undoubtedly our
primeval ancestors. Many of the physical attributes of cattle ren-
dered them unsuitable for domestication, in particular their large
size and the low proportion of muscle tissues in the areas giving
desirable meat cuts, such as the loin. However, aspects of cattle
behaviour and their ability to thrive on grasses of little value to man
led early man to choose cattle as the major domesticated animal.
Their limited agility, gregarious social structure, the promiscuity of
the male and extrovert receptivity display by the female, as well as
the precocial development of the young, are probably responsible for
the relative ease with which they must have entered into a sym-
biotic relationship with man. This led to their domestication and the
development of mutual respect for the benefits that each brought to
the other.

Nowadays the study of cattle behaviour is no less important. They
are still our major domesticated animal, contributing worldwide
almost 18% of man's protein intake and 9% of our energy intake, as
well as draught power, hides and dung for fuel. In the increasing
pressure to intensify cattle production, it is often forgotten that the
unit in the factory production system is a higher mammal, with
complex mental and physical needs. The reaction of cattle to a
production system is best overtly observed in terms of their behavioural response. The animal's physiological response can also be
measured and may be closely related to its production rate but
usually bears little relationship to its behaviour and to the adequacy
of the environment. The latter is best indicated by the animal's
behaviour, both the ability to display normal behaviour patterns and
the absence of abnormal, deleterious behaviour. For humans an

animal's behaviour is a signal about its well-being; for cattle it is the reaction to the environment as they perceive it, modified by the innate motivation to perform the behaviours.

Veterinarians utilise cattle behavioural signals for disease diagnosis, and livestock handlers on the farm can also derive useful information on the health of the stock in their charge from their behaviour.

This book attempts to describe the major behaviour patterns in cattle, their ontogeny and in particular their purpose. It is intended for farmers and stockpeople, students of agriculture, veterinary medicine and ethology and it is hoped that it will be of interest to advisers in cattle husbandry and cattle researchers.

CLIVE PHILLIPS
Bangor, Gwynedd

ACKNOWLEDGEMENTS

I am grateful to the many people who have given me encouragement and support during the long gestation period of this book. In particular I owe much to staff and research students at the University College of North Wales, Bangor for their help in my research of cattle behaviour, especially Professor J. B. Owen, Dr S. A. Schofield, Dr S. E. Kitwood, Dr P. C. Chiy, Dr M. Youssef, Dr H. Omed, Dr N. L. James, Mr L. Weiguo, Mr T. Arab, Mr K. Hecheimi, Mr J. Pilling, Mr J. M. Owen and Mr J. Ffridd.

I am grateful for permission from various sources to reproduce copyright material in tables and figures. Full documentation is given in the reference lists at the end of each chapter. While attempts have been made to secure permission for all material bound by copyright, we have been unable to trace some copyright holders. Acknowledgements will be given in later editions if the copyright holders contact Farming Press.

I am also grateful to those who have helped directly in the production of the book: to Mrs G. Owen for typing most of it, to Mr R. Smith and Mrs J. Arnold of Farming Press for their patience and assistance, to Mr D. Piggins for reading and commenting on Chapter 1 and not least to my wife and children for their support throughout.

CP

CHAPTER 1

ENVIRONMENTAL PERCEPTION

An animal's behaviour is its reaction to stimuli and this is modified by its perception of the internal and external environment. The internal environment is created largely by endogenous rhythms, which generate motivation but are influenced by exogenous circumstances. The external environment is perceived through sensory faculties, especially the five classical senses of sight, taste, touch, hearing, olfaction. Other environmental phenomena are perceived, such as gravitational forces and the weather, and, though generally of less importance, may at times strongly influence behaviour. Signals provided by the sensory receptors, often embedded in specialised organs, are then processed by the brain to produce information that can be acted upon and memorised if necessary. Farm animals differ from humans in both their sensory and processing capacities, and a more detailed knowledge of this information, and the use to which it is put, is essential if we are to understand the animal's interaction with its environment.

VISION

Some of the major senses are used relatively infrequently, but vision is involved to some extent in the perception of most stimuli and has been shown, as in humans, to be the dominant sense in many situations (Blaschke *et al.*, 1984) and to be responsible for approximately 50% of total sensory information. Aspects of visual information processing can be estimated by optometric measurements of the eye (e.g. radius of curvature, refractive power), by measuring neuronal activity in the visual cortex of the brain or by investigating the behaviour of the animal psychophysically.

1

Animals are thought to obtain visual information in three stages (Figure 1.1). Initially a primal sketch is formed from the retinal images; then from this is extracted the information relevant to, for example, depth, motion, shape, size and shadow, which is processed to form a stereoscopic image. Finally there is abstraction in combination with cognitive memory to produce information that can be stored and/or acted upon. In farm animals stage one—primal sketch formation—is undoubtedly similar to that in humans because of the similarity of eye structure. Cattle have both rod and cone receptors, with 2–3 rods per cone in the fovea and 5–6 near the papilla. This suggests a good mechanism for colour vision and it has been confirmed psychophysically that cattle can discriminate colour well (Gilbert and Arave, 1986; Riol et al., 1989), especially at long wavelengths (yellow, orange and red). The ability for animals like cattle that were once prey to perceive red accurately and respond rapidly may reflect its survival value when a member of the herd was attacked and blood appeared. This feature of cattle vision may be utilised when bullfighters provide a red stimuli for the bull to charge.

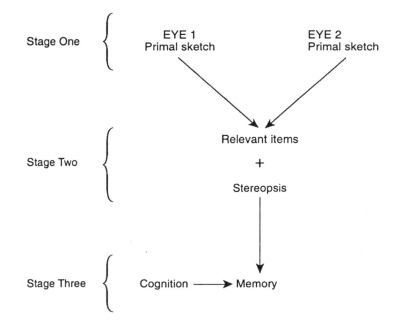

Figure 1.1. Visual information collection and processing.

Some difficulty is experienced by cattle in distinguishing blue, grey and green (the shorter wavelengths) (Riol *et al.*, 1989), but sheep are known to be able to select grass that is dark green rather than light green. Possibly light intensity rather than hue is the cue used here, although cattle have less ability to discriminate light intensity than humans (Figure 1.2). Cattle also have limited power of lens accommodation—changing the shape of the lens to allow focusing to take place. In considering the second stage, shape discrimination powers are high in cattle (Baldwin, 1981), suggesting both fairly good visual acuity and synthesis of information from stage one.

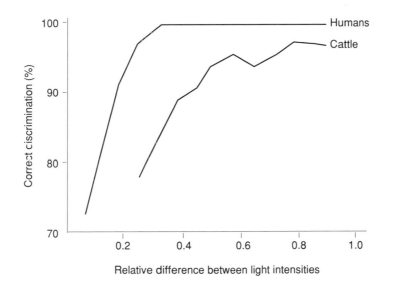

Figure 1.2   Light intensity discrimination capabilities of humans and cattle. *(Phillips and Weiguo, 1990)*

Another limitation of the bovine eye is the restricted amount of binocular vision that is possible (Figure 1.3). Eyes are positioned on the side of the head to give a good field of vision, about 330° in cattle, which is good for predator awareness. In animals free from predation, eyes are generally positioned towards or at the front of the head, man for example possessing only 180° visual field. The limited overlap of ruminant eyes, only 30–50° compared to 140° in man,

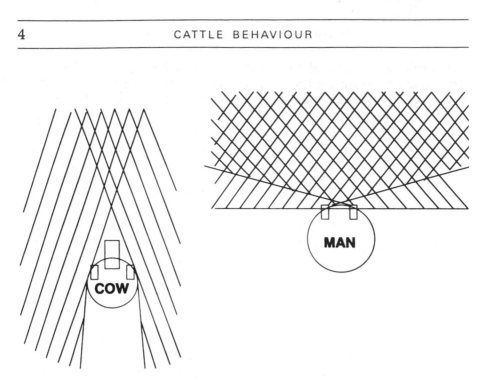

Figure 1.3 Overlap in the human and bovine visual fields.

means that stereoscopic vision is probably limited at short distances, depending on the position of the fovea. However, other means are employed to judge distance: moving objects can be positioned by overlap of monocular cues (parallax), and memory of object size will allow distance to be estimated. 'Danger' recognition is therefore more likely if the subject is moving and can be recognised and related to previous experience.

In addition to receiving and conveying information on visual images, the photic stimulus is also used to set the internal clock of the animal. Perception of photoperiod appears to be relative rather than absolute, since there are strong residual effects of photoperiod in lighting manipulation experiments. Cattle can be 'tricked' into producing the physiological response to a long day by supplementing a 6 hour light period with a burst of light for 15–60 minutes in the middle of the dark period. Probably they have a photosensitive period about 15–18 hours after dawn. Although diurnal rhythms are evident in the absence of photoperiodic cues, the light:dark cycle is responsible for fine-tuning the clock.

In cattle the length of the light cycle also has specific effects on reproduction (to match the peak intake requirement of offspring to peak feed availability) and production. Cattle probably perceive both changes in photoperiod and actual photoperiod. Least productivity is obtained from cows in a declining, short daylength. Behaviour is also affected as a high light:dark ratio reduces aggression and locomotion in adverse environments (Weiguo and Phillips, 1991). The latter may be related to a feedback of prolactin on the hypothalamus, causing neurones to increase dopamine synthesis (Zinn et al., 1989). Certainly cattle will work for a light reward, and the preference is for a daylength of approximately 16 hours (Baldwin and Start, 1981), which has also been shown to give the highest productivity compared with 10 or 24 hour daylengths.

HEARING

Although hearing tends to be of less importance and is less researched in cattle than vision, it is of particular importance in inter- and intra-species communication. The mammalian ear shows little species diversity, but even so human auditory discrimination powers are generally greater than those of other animals, perhaps because of the greater complexity of human vocal communication.

The audible range of frequencies is, however, more restricted in humans than cattle. Optimum frequency (the point at which a sound can be heard with the least amplitude or volume) occurs at about 1–4 kHz in humans and at 8 kHz in cattle, and here the intensity threshold is lowest at about 26 decibels (Heffner and Heffner, 1983). This 'best frequency' is usually reserved for the overtones of high-frequency alarm calls, which in cattle reach 8 kHz. Below this intensity the hearing threshold increases, i.e. the sound has to be louder to be heard, and the minimum frequency that can be detected by humans and cattle is similar at 20–25 Hz (Figure 1.4). Above 8 kHz the hearing threshold increases again, and the maximum intensity that can be perceived is 35 kHz in cattle but only 20 kHz in humans. The high-frequency hearing limit is generally related to the inter-aural distance: mammals with a large interaural distance, such as the elephant, have a reduced high-frequency hearing limit (Figure 1.5). However, cattle have a similar interaural distance to that of humans but a much greater high-frequency hearing limit (Heffner and Masterton, 1990). This may relate to the need for cattle to be able to hear small predators, such as vampire bats (*Desmodus rotundus*), that use high-frequency vocalisations. On hearing the call of the

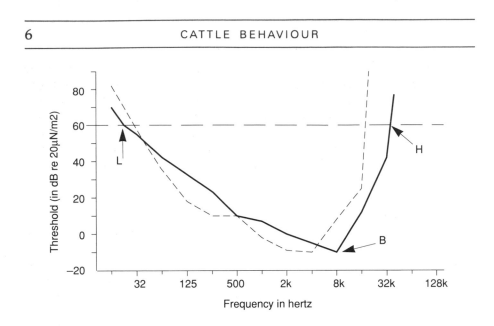

Figure 1.4   Hearing curve in cattle (———) and humans (– – –). For cattle B = best hearing frequency; H = high frequency hearing limit; L = low frequency hearing limit. (Heffner and Masterton, 1990)

vampire bat, cattle will flee and disperse to an open area where bats are unlikely to attack (Delpietro, 1989). Humans, despite popular legend, rarely get attacked by vampire bats, although this can occur if the bats get caught in a person's hair, the neck being an obvious target area of flesh. High-pitched sounds, such as from parlour machinery, may disturb cattle but not be audible to man. In summary, cattle have less ability than humans to detect small differences between sound frequencies, though they possess a greater audible frequency range.

A second aspect of hearing—binaural localisation—relates to the animal's ability to position a sound accurately, in the same way that binocular vision enables the accurate distance of a visual stimulus to be determined. Many animals have this ability to locate the direction of a sound accurately, at least in the vertical plane. Animals are generally less able to judge sound direction in the horizontal plane or to judge the distance over which a sound has travelled before it reaches them. There are two mechanisms that can be used for sound localisation in the vertical plane. First, differences in the phase of the sound as it arrives at the two ears, which is used to locate low-frequency tones, and secondly, differences in the frequency of the sound between the two ears, which serves better to locate high-frequency tones. Both cattle and man would be expected to have a small sound localisation threshold because of their large inter-aural distance (Figure 1.5). However, whereas humans use both mechanisms to be able to accurately locate a sound to within 1°, cattle use mainly intensity difference cues and can only locate a sound to within 30°.

This may relate to the fact that, from an evolutionary standpoint, it was more important for predators, such as man, to be able to pinpoint the direction of their prey, whereas prey animals, such as cattle, need only a rough idea of where danger lies before fleeing. Some animals, such as man, that have a strong fovea to give good visual acuity in the centre of their field of vision also need to reinforce this with accurate sound localisation, whereas cattle with a weak fovea and a broad field of best vision do not need this degree of accuracy. There are also good physiological reasons for believing that animals with poor binocular vision will have poor binaural localisation powers.

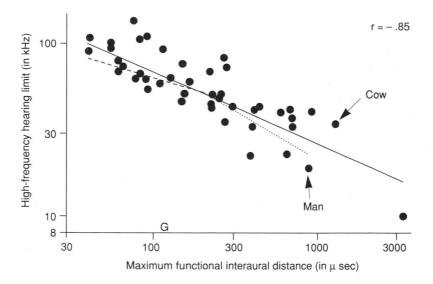

Figure 1.5　Relation between maximum functional interaural distance (interaural distance/speed of sound) and the highest audible frequency (at 60 db SPL) for the more than 40 mammals with complete behavioural audiograms. (H ffner and Masterton, 1990)

OLFACTION

Despite man's bizarre insistence on masking, replacing or removing his own olfactory signals, these are generally of extreme importance in intra-species communication in cattle, and rank with vision as a prime sensing mechanism. In particular they are important in the synchronisation and advancement of reproduction, in territorial marking and for signalling predators.

Unlike humans, who smell only through the nasal organ, there are two major sites of odour reception in cattle—the nose and the vomeronasal or Jacobson's organ, the latter being primarily used for social communication. This organ is situated in the roof of the mouth and consists of blind tubular diverticula lined with olfactory epithelium. Air is sampled via the buccal cavity and the nose although the nostrils are partially closed by the lip curling in this behaviour. The characteristic flehman expression, whereby the head is directed upwards with the mouth ajar, the tongue flat and the upper lips curled back (Plate 1.1) is thought to aid odour sampling in ruminants by allowing air to be inhaled so that it passes over the roof of the mouth.

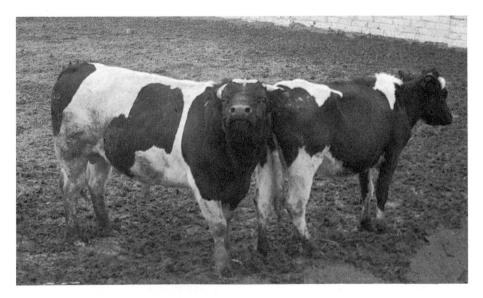

Plate 1.1   Flehman expression in a bull guarding a cow.

There is no evidence for chemical selectivity of the organ, but as with the nose a wide range of volatile aerosol chemicals can be detected. The chemical sensitivity of cattle ranges from being able to detect very weak solutions of sodium salts up to large hydrocarbon molecules and steroids (Bell and Sly, 1983). Thus cattle are able to detect odours from inanimate and animate objects and utilize the information to modify their reproductive, ingestive or social behaviour.

Pheromones are a specialised group of chemical attractants produced by animals to stimulate other animals. They are present in all body fluids including sweat, and there are many different types in cattle including alcohols, diols, alkanes, ethers, diethers, ketones, primary amines and aromatic alkanes. The specific oestrous odours are probably released from the body surface, particularly the hindquarters and genital region, rather than urine, faeces or vaginal mucus (Blazquez *et al.*, 1988).

In comparison with man, a microsmatic animal, cattle are macrosmatic. Although specific tests have not been conducted for cattle, they can almost certainly detect much smaller differences in odour concentration than man can. For example, man can usually detect an intensity difference about one-third that of the actual intensity, whereas rodents can detect a difference of one-twenty-fifth. Some divergence of olfactory apparatus occurs in cattle, e.g. in sexual attraction the nose is used for preliminary diagnosis of oestrous odours and the vomeronasal organ is used for reinforcement and the maintenance of sexual interest during copulation. Flehman is also believed to act for appeasement, being the antithesis of the threat display. In deer, but not sheep, smell is also important in diet selection. Although specific tests have not been conducted with cattle, it is likely that smell is unimportant for cattle grazing a uniform pasture with a limited range of botanical species, because repeated exposure to odour stimuli reduces sensitivity as the receptor sites become locked up.

In humans smell perception may be impaired not so much by the sensory apparatus as by the information processing by the brain. However, although many people are not aware of it, humans are able to identify their own odours, synchronise menstrual cycles using body odours and recognise their mothers' odour at 5 days of age.

TASTE

Chemoreception by taste (gustation) has been extensively studied in man and cattle. Generally four primary tastes are identifiable and can be correlated to physiological requirements: sweet for nutrient supply, salt to control electrolyte balance, bitter to avoid toxins, and sour to regulate pH. There may also be separate metallic and monosodium glutamate tastes, but probably all tastes derive from combinations of signals from these four primary taste receptors. The receptors are located in specific areas of the tongue, and differ in their taste discrimination, sensitivity and positioning on the tongue between cattle and man. In man the tip of the tongue is sensitive to sweet and salt taste, but in cattle sweet taste is mainly at the base and salt at the tip (Hard *et al.*, 1989). The reason for this is unclear but the increased use of the base of the tongue for gustatory signals in cattle may arise from the longer period of time that food is masticated in the middle to rear section of the buccal cavity compared with man.

Several compounds that taste sweet to man, e.g. monellin and thaumartin, do not elicit a response in cattle. Cattle generally experience a greater sweet taste from monosaccharides than disaccharides, with the most potent sweeteners being glycine, Na-saccharin and xylintol. When presented with NaCl, xylintol also enhances the salt taste. The bovine tongue is not very receptive to quinine, which has a strong, bitter taste to humans.

There are also no distinct water receptors in cattle as there are in man, but the posterior part of the bovine tongue is responsive to material flow, using mechanoreceptors, and can detect water passage. Thermoreceptors are also present in the tongue. The regurgitated bolus provides a mechanism for chemoreception of rumen conditions, especially acidity.

Taste perception develops at an early age in ruminants. It has been shown to develop in the sheep foetus in mid pregnancy, and maternal diet can possibly affect dietary preferences of juveniles through *in utero* influences. Taste perception and discrimination thresholds change with advancing age. In cattle the discrimination threshold to sucrose is less for calves than adult cows. In sheep the intensity of salt flavour ascribed to a standard NaCl solution increases fourfold from the foetus to adulthood, whereas that to KCl decreases by about 30%. Adult cattle prefer pure water to a 0.09 NaCl solution but calves do not, suggesting that a similar increase in NaCl perception with age occurs in cattle as in sheep. KCl is a less potent salt flavour than NaCl in cattle.

EPIDERMAL RECEPTORS

The skin contains a number of sensory receptors, particularly mechanoreceptors to detect movement and force, thermoreceptors to detect temperature and nociceptors to detect damaging stimuli and pathological conditions, such as inflammation. These are more numerous in the sensitive areas of the body—in cattle, for example, the lips, tongue, nose, udder and vulval labia. Humans have increased sensitivity in the hands, especially the fingertips, which effectively become sampling tools in exploratory situations. Ungulates do not have this facility and frequently use their extended buccal protrusion for this purpose.

NOCICEPTION AND PAIN

All the evidence suggests that cattle have a similar neural mechanism to humans (Iggo, 1984). The emotional response to noxious stimuli increases with the magnitude and degree of novelty of the stimuli (Stephens and Jones, 1975). The presence of herdmates reduces the emotional response, and there is some evidence of difference between species. In many circumstances the response to pain and possibly pain perception itself is not as great in cattle as in man, which may be because cattle were prey animals and man was a predator. It is usually disadvantageous for a prey animal to indicate that it is in pain, as it may be singled out for attack by a predator. However, higher-order predators such as man are more likely to benefit from a pain response, particularly high-frequency vocalisation (an alarm call) to attract assistance and divert the mind from an excessive (shock) reaction.

Pain suppression may be mediated through endogenously secreted opioids. The analgesic opioids are antinociceptive agents that appear to raise the threshold for pain perception and act on the same part of the brain that morphine affects. Thus one such agent—beta endorphin, an endogenous morphine-like substance—is believed to allow the passive reception of highly noxious stimuli in both cattle and man, with little perception of pain, partly to avoid a damaging adrenal reaction and possibly in cattle also to avoid attracting predators.

A further reason for reduced pain response in cattle may be that, although there can be little doubt that they do feel pain, the cerebral capacity to process information from nociceptors and produce painful sensations from it may be less than in humans (Iggo, 1984). It is the cerebral cortex that processes sensory stimuli and this region of the brain is much more developed in man than in cattle. This does not necessarily mean that cattle feel less pain than humans, but may indicate that they suffer less psychologically from the long-term consequences of pain—anxiety, depression, etc. It should be remembered that the size of an organ may have little relation to its perceptive ability—people with large noses do not necessarily have greater olfactory powers—and behavioural studies do not necessarily support this theory.

REFERENCES

Baldwin, B. A., and Start, B. 1981. 'Sensory reinforcement and illumination preference in sheep and calves.' *Proceedings of the Royal Society, London,* B211, 513–526.

Baldwin, B. A. 1981. 'Shape discrimination in sheep and calves.' *Animal Behaviour,* 29, 830–834.

Bell, F. R., and Sly, J. 1983. 'The olfactory detection of sodium and lithium salts by sodium deficient cattle.' *Physiology and Behaviour,* 31, 307–312.

Blaschke, C. F., Thompson, D. L., Humes, P. E., and Godke, R. A. 1984. 'Olfaction, sight and auditory perception of mature bulls in detecting estrual responses in beef heifers.' *Proceedings of the 10th International Congress on Animal Reproduction and Artificial Insemination,* 10–14 June 1984. Paper 284, 3 pp. University of Illinois, Urbana, USA.

Blazques, N. B., French, J. M., Lang, S. E., and Perry, G. C. 1988. 'A phenomenal function for the perineal skin glands in the cow.' *Veterinary Record,* 123, 49–50.

Delpietro, H. A. 1989. 'Case reports on defensive behaviour in equine and bovine subjects in response to vocalisations of the common vampire bat (Desmodus rotundus).' *Applied Animal Behaviour Science,* 22, 377–380.

Gilbert, B. J., and Arave, C. W. 1986. 'Ability of cattle to distinguish among different wavelengths of light.' *Journal of Dairy Science,* 69, 825–832.

Hard, C. A. F., Segerstad, A. F., and Hellekant, G. 1989. 'The sweet taste in the calf.' *Physiology and Behaviour,* 45, 633–638 and 1043–1047.

Heffner, R. S., and Heffner, H. E. 1983. 'Hearing in large mammals: Horses (Equus caballus) and cattle (Bos taurus).' *Behavioural Neuroscience,* 97, 299–309.

Heffner, R. S., and Masterton, R. B. 1990. 'Sound localisation in mammals: brain-stem mechanisms.' In *Comparative Perception, Vol. 1. Basic Mechanism* (ed. Berkley, M. A., and Stebbins, W. C.). John Wiley and Sons, Inc.

Iggo, A. 1984. 'Pain in animals.' Hume Memorial lecture, 15 November 1984. University Federation for Animal Welfare, London.

Phillips, C. J. C., and Weiguo, L. 1991. 'Brightness discrimination abilities of calves relative to that of humans.' *Applied Animal Behaviour Science*, 31, 25–33.

Riol, J. A., Sanchez, J. M., Egwen, U. G., and Gaudioso, U. R. 1989. 'Colour perception in fighting cattle.' *Applied Animal Behaviour Science*, 23, 199–208.

Stephens, D. B., and Jones, J. N. 1975. 'Husbandry influences on some physiological parameters of emotional responses in calves.' *Applied Animal Ethology*, 1, 233–243.

Weiguo, L., and Phillips, C. J. C. 1991. 'The effects of supplementary light on the behaviour and performance of calves.' *Applied Animal Behaviour Science*, 30, 27–34.

Zinn, S. A., Chapin, L. T., Lookingland, K. J., Moore, K. E., and Tucker, H. A. 1989. 'Effects of photoperiod on tuberoinfundibular dopaminergic (TIDA) nerone aid on lactotropes in Holstein bull calves.' *Journal of Dairy Science*, 72, supplt. 1, 338–339.

CHAPTER 2

ACQUISITION OF BEHAVIOUR

INNATE OR LEARNT?

For a long time scientists have been unsure how much behaviour is inherited genetically and how much is learnt through environmental experience. One way to resolve this is to look at the behaviour of animals isolated from the relevant environmental influences at birth. Even this is of dubious validity for some behaviours; for example with vocalization there is evidence that animals can learn the sound of their mother's call in the womb. Even so, there is no doubt that some behaviours, particularly those needed immediately after birth, are entirely innate (fully developed and complete at first appearance). Examples of these are suckling and standing and those rhythmical behaviours which are fundamental to the life process (and tend to be under the control of the autonomic nervous system) such as breathing, defecation, etc. Experiments where cows have been reared in isolation as calves have shown them to be socially maladjusted as adults—less dominant, more nervous, less interactive with other cows and having poor mothering ability (Warnick *et al.*, 1977).

Learning evolves from a motivation to acquire information through experience. It is more rapid in young cattle, but they also forget quickest (Kovalcikova and Kovalcik, 1984). For example the rudiments of sexual behaviour are inherited and possibly the motivation, but the successful operator has to learn the fine art of courtship display, mounting, etc. Most complex behaviours, particularly those not used in early life such as sexual behaviour, have an element of learning involved. Inexperienced bulls in particular show a high degree of unsuccessful mounts, many of which are head to head or head to side. Mastering the mounting process takes place not only through operant conditioning of mature cattle but also

15

during the play process.

Some behaviours are acquired solely through the learning process, and these include many of the activities cattle are required to perform under the control of man, e.g. operating an out-of-parlour feeding device. These activities have to be learnt, because genetic selection for these behaviours has not occurred in the limited time that cattle have existed in man's intensive husbandry system. They may be learnt directly from man himself, as when calves are trained to drink milk from buckets, or from fellow herdmates, which is increasingly necessary as herds increase in size and the time for human contact between man and individual animals is limited.

This is not to say that man has had no influence on the genetic control of cattle behaviour. Culling of animals with difficult temperament has almost certainly contributed to the docility of cows today, and the improved reproductive performance of cows exhibiting strong homosexual oestrous activity has probably enhanced this characteristic (Baker and Seidel, 1975).

HERITABILITIES OF BEHAVIOUR

Few experiments have been conducted to estimate the genetic, as opposed to environmental effects on behaviour traits (Table 2.1). The inheritance of feeding behaviour was first studied scientifically by Hancock (1950) using monozygotic twin dairy cows. This work suggested a strong genetic component to grazing behaviour, although environmental effects could not be totally disregarded. Later research (Macha and Olsarova, 1986), however, has shown weak inheritance of grazing behaviour.

Grazing behaviour and feeding behaviour with conserved feeds appear not to be highly correlated, because the ingestive behaviour of cattle offered conserved feeds is highly heritable but for grazing cattle it is not (Baehr et al., 1984; Mokhov, 1983). Probably there has been less natural selection for feeding on conserved fodder than for long grazing times. This may be because cows are short of time to consume sufficient grazed herbage (see Chapter 5), but not to eat sufficient conserved feeds because of the higher rate of ingestion. There are obvious advantages for cattle that are prepared to graze for a long time, at the expense of other behaviours such as resting, and there has probably been natural selection for this trait. A second factor is that selection for grazing time could have occurred gradually over many millenia, whereas cattle have been given conserved feeds by man for only a very limited period.

TABLE 2.1 Heritability estimates of behavioural traits. Heritability range is from 0.01, weakly inherited, to 0.3+, strongly inherited.

	Behaviour	Heritability
PERSONALITY		
O'Bleness *et al.*, 1960	Temperament	0.40 ± 0.09
New Zealand Dairy Board, 1961	Temperament	0.06
Beilharz *et al.*, 1966	Dominance	0.44
Dickson *et al.*, 1970	Temperament	0.53
Shrode and Hammock, 1971	Temperament	0.40 ± 0.30
Brown, 1974	Maternal protective temperament	0.32 (Hereford) 0.17 (Angus)
Mishra *et al.*, 1975	Temperament	0.19
Persson, 1978	Temperament	0.12 – 0.18 0.16 – 0.45 0.24
Salcido and Eugenio, 1979	Temperament	0.04
Wickham, 1979	Temperament	0.11
Stricklin *et al.*, 1980	Temperament	0.48 ± 0.29
Sato, 1981	Temperament	0.45 – 0.67
Agyemang *et al.*, 1982	Disposition (degree of trouble to herdsman)	0.03
Fordyce *et al.*, 1982	Movement in crush	0.25 ± 0.20
	Movement in race	0.17 ± 0.21
	Movement in crush plus head restraint	0.67 ± 0.26
	Audible respiration in crush	0.20 ± 0.16
	Audible respiration in race	0.57 ± 0.22
Mokhov, 1983	Cattle encounters	0.52
	Cattle aggressive interactions	0.88
Baehr *et al.*, 1984	Quiet behaviour	0.75 ± 0.38
	Fast movement	0.61 ± 0.38
Fordyce and Goddard, 1984	Temperament in crush	0.0 – 0.10*
	Vigour of movement	0.0
	Audible respiration	0.0
	Kicking	0.0
	Bellowing	0.09
	Kneeling down	0.10

(*Continued*)

TABLE 2.1 (*Continued*)

	Behaviour	Heritability
Hearnshaw and Morris, 1984	Temperament	0.03 ± 0.28 (B. taurus) 0.46 ± 0.37 (B. indicus)
Buddenberg et al., 1986	Maternal behaviour (protection of calf from humans)	0.06 ± 0.01
INGESTIVE BEHAVIOUR		
Mokhov, 1983	Feeding duration	0.68
	Ruminating duration	0.59
Baehr et al., 1984	Visits to concentrate dispenser	0.61 ± 0.27
Macha and Olsarova, 1986	Grazing time per day	0.003 ± 0.026
Santha et al., 1988	Rumination time per day	0.15
	Rumination bout length	0.20
Mendoza-Ordones et al., 1988	Drinking rate	0.43
	Gulps per second	0.68
	Intake per gulp	0.52
REPRODUCTIVE BEHAVIOUR		
Rottensten and Touchberry, 1957	Oestrous intensity	0.21
Blockey et al., 1978	Serving capacity	0.59 ± 0.16

* Significant dam-daughter correlations, suggesting a non-genetic maternal effect.

The other major behavioural characteristic to be examined for genetic influence is personality. This has been measured both as the behavioural response of cows with calves to approach by humans and as the behaviour of cattle in a confinement crush. The response of a cow with calf to humans has a low to moderate heritability and a low genetic correlation with production characteristics. Temperament in the crush has generally been found to have a variable heritability of 0–0.4. However, greater heritabilities have been found when cattle are highly challenged in the crush by imposition of a head restraint. Greater heritabilities have also been found in *Bos indicus* cattle, which are generally more difficult to handle than *Bos taurus*. This suggests that an extreme nervous reaction or 'fit' in the crush is more highly heritable than the normal range of reactions seen during mild stress in the crush. Undoubtedly there has been prolonged selection by humans for resistance to milking stress, but possibly not for a major stress reaction such as some animals exhibit in a crush. Repeatability of temperament scores in the crush has generally been high, suggesting that measurement technique is not a problem, although the different aspects of temperament—movement, respiration, bellowing, kicking—that have been recorded to represent temperament might account for some of the variation in results.

These results show that, despite inconsistencies, the heritability of some behaviours is high, particularly those that have not been selected for before or during domestication. We might expect a low heritability for reproductive behaviour, where it is related to reproductive potential, because of the obvious survival value of this behaviour in the past. Similarly we would expect docility to have been selected for during the process of domestication and still to be selected for today. In contrast, behaviours associated with the use of man-made equipment, such as concentrate dispensers, will not have been selected for and tend to have a high heritability. A few behavioural traits have also been linked to major genes, such as fearfulness in double-muscled cattle, but most are assumed to be multigene traits.

METHODS OF LEARNING

Operant Conditioning

This form of learning evolves from obtaining a desirable (reward) status when a certain action in exploration of the environment is taken. It is effectively trial and error learning, in that it is necessary for the animal to experience the reward repeatedly before the behaviour is learnt. For example, a cow learning to use an out-of-parlour feeder eventually learns that if she puts her head in the reception area, feed is delivered into the trough. All animals are programmed to be inquisitive to a certain degree so that they can take advantage of new opportunities arising in the environment.

Operant conditioning is the most common form of learning in cattle since they are not timid animals and will readily explore new situations. The mechanism can be a powerful tool for a researcher in learning about cattle's perception of the environment.

Classical Conditioning

This form of conditioning is distinct from trial and error learning in that it involves the formation of an association between an unrelated 'neutral' stimulus and a response. The response is 'conditioned' once this association is formed. The classic example is Pavlov's dog, which was trained to salivate when a tuning fork was sounded, because this was associated with the provision of meat as a reward. Subsequently, the dog salivated whether or not the meat was provided, although in time the response became extinguished as the dog learnt that the association had been broken.

Most learning in farm animals is initially by trial and error but the response is maintained through the formation of associations between one or more neutral stimuli and the response. Cattle kept in confinement are usually in a precise rhythm of behaviour patterns and they soon learn to distinguish the sequence of events that precedes the direct stimulation of a response. For example, a wagon delivering feed in a cattle shed normally elicits immediate feeding behaviour, but may be preceded by the sight or sound of the man starting a tractor, putting feed into the feeder wagon or simply opening the door to the shed. These neutral stimuli are then more likely to elicit the feeding response than the later conditioned stimulus, particularly in a competitive situation where the first cows to the feeding barrier get the most feed.

Animals use the simplest and most reliable stimuli to elicit a response. If they had to interpret all the signals before they responded, it would be a waste of their energy and they would be slow to act. So they only use a small number of stimuli and often only one aspect of each. The bright red colour of the tractor that will feed them may be sufficient if this is the only time they encounter it. Similarly, dairy cows are thought to be initially operant conditioned to letdown their milk as they find that allowing the cluster to be put on their udder releases the pressure. Soon, however, the response becomes classically conditioned and the cows use conditioned stimuli, such as entry to the collecting yard, to trigger milk letdown.

Conditioned learning can be a powerful tool to learn about the discrimination powers of animals. For instance, calves placed at the entrance to two chambers, one of which had a brighter light source than the other, were able to learn how to indicate the correct chamber in order to receive a feed reward. Their discrimination power can be detected and compared to other species by varying the difference between the lights. It must be remembered, however, that it takes a long time to train calves to perform such activities. In this case (Phillips and Weiguo, 1991) it took 40 tests before correct discrimination of widely differing light sources could be achieved and the discrimination power test could begin (Figure 2.1). The information obtained must be combined with anatomical and behavioural observation to get a more complete idea of discrimination power. Usually a feed reward is provided for making a correct discrimination in these tests, but in some instances very precise positioning of the animal is required, e.g. to test binaural localisation powers (see Chapter 1), and the 'reward' for correct discrimination may have to be the avoidance of a mild electric shock.

Conditioned learning can also be used to train cattle to indicate their preferences, and the strength of (or motivation for) these preferences is shown by pushing a lever. The lever is usually

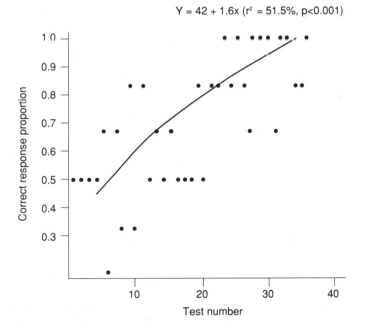

Figure 2.1 Learning curve of calves during the training period of a light intensity discrimination test.

mounted about 1m from the floor, or alternatively the animal may break a beam passing between two photoelectric cells. The animal can receive such rewards as feed or light by the lever or beam. However, it is difficult to distinguish a definite preference from the animal playing with the activator. This may be partially overcome by comparing the activation of the lever or beam with a dummy lever or beam, which produces no response. Alternatively the number of lever presses required to elicit the response can be increased (fixed ratio schedule) or the period of time that elapses between lever pressing and the response increased (fixed interval schedule). Introducing a cost to the animal (work for the fixed ratio schedule, time for the fixed interval schedule) allows the researcher to determine to what extent the animal is motivated to receive the reward.

Insight learning

The more complex an animal's behaviour, the more it needs to store stimuli–response details and use these to control behaviour. Most higher-order animals can put together a sequence of these response patterns to produce a required response.

For example, a cow will go through an elaborate procedure of bullying a less dominant cow at an individual concentrate feeder in order to evict her and get access herself to the residue of the concentrate portion. The complexity of the tasks that will be performed to achieve a result may give some indication of the intelligence of the animals, but it is also related to the degree of exploratory behaviour they perform. More nervous and less exploratory cattle are slower to learn conditioned responses.

Investigatory behaviour

Investigatory behaviour is clearly at the heart of much of learning. It is most common in the young calf, but this is likely to be partly because the number of new stimuli are very high at this time, and as the calf gets accustomed to its environment, less exploratory behaviour is produced.

The posture of cattle exploring the environment displays the degree of confidence that they have in the response. A confident approach is one where the head is not greatly extended (colour plate 1), whereas an unconfident approach allows for a more rapid retreat by extending the head (containing the sensory organs) further and keeping a greater distance between the stimulus and the means of retreat, the legs (Plate 2.1).

Tests of learning ability in cattle have been numerous, including a

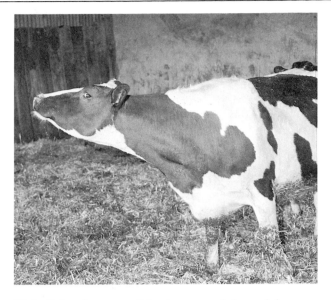

Plate 2.1 An unconfident approach by a dairy cow.

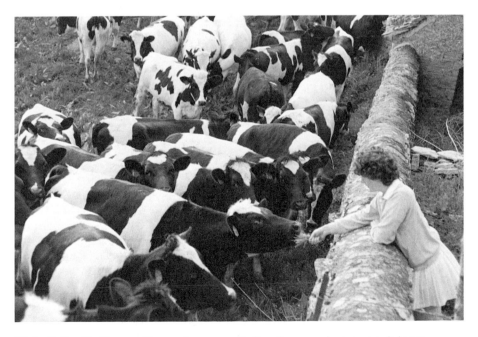

Plate 2.2 Cattle readily explore novel situations and as a result learn quickly.

multiple choice selection (Gardner, 1937), training to do specific tasks (Breland and Breland, 1966) and even performance in mazes (Kilgour, 1981). Perhaps not surprisingly, Kilgour found that cattle performed better than cats and opossums in a maze since they readily explore new areas (Plate 2.2) and in particular move into open spaces, whereas many other species tend to 'hug the walls' of the maze and take longer to complete the operation.

REFERENCES

Agyemang, K., Clapp, E., and Van Vleck, L. D. 1982. 'Components of variance of dairymen's workability traits among Holstein cows.' *Journal of Dairy Science*, 65, 1334–1338.

Baehr, J., Schulte-Coerne, H. , Pabst, K. , Gravert, H. O. 1984. (The behaviour of cows in cubicles). *Zuchtungskunde* 56, 127–138.

Baker, A. E. M., and Seidel, G. E. 1975. 'Why do cows mount other cows?' *Applied Animal Behaviour Science*, 13, 237–241.

Beilharz, R. G., Butcher, D. F., and Freeman, A. E. 1966. 'Social dominance and milk production in Holsteins.' *Journal of Dairy Science*, 49, 887–892.

Blockey, M. A. de. B., Straw, W. M., and Jones, L. P. 1978. 'Heritability of serving capacity and scrotal circumference in beef bulls.' *70th Annual Meeting Abstracts*, American Society of Animal Science, 253.

Breland, K., and Breland, M. 1966. *Animal Behaviour*. Macmillan, New York.

Brown, W. G. Jr. 1974. 'Some aspects of beef cattle behaviour as related to productivity.' *Dissertation Abstracts International* B, 34, 1805.

Buddenberg, B. J., Brown, C. J., Johnson, Z. B., and Honea, R. S. 1986. 'Maternal behaviour of beef cows at parturition.' *Journal of Animal Science*, 62, 42–46.

Dickson, D. P., Barr, G. R., and Wieckert, D. A. 1967. 'Social relationships of dairy cows in a feed lot.' *Behaviour*, 29, 196–203.

Fordyce, G., and Goddard, M. E. 1984. 'Maternal influence on the temperament of Bos indicus cross cows.' *Proceedings of the Australian Society of Animal Production*, 15, 345–348.

Fordyce, G., Goddard, M. E., and Seifert, G. W. 1982. The measurement of temperament in cattle and the effect of genotype and experience. *Proceedings of the Australian Society of Animal Production*, 14, 329–332.

Gardner, L. P. 1937. 'The response of cows in a discrimination problem.' *Journal of Comparative Psychology*, 23, 35–37.

Hancock, J. 1950. 'Studies in monozygotic cattle twins. IV Uniformity trials: grazing behaviour.' *New Zealand Journal of Science and Technology* A, 32, 22–59.

Hearnshaw, H., and Morris, C. A. 1984. 'Genetic and environmental effects on a temperament score in beef cattle.' *Australian Journal of Agricultural Research*, 35, 723–773.

Kilgour, R. 1981. 'Use of the Hebb-Williams closed field test to study the learning ability of Jersey cows.' *Animal Behaviour*, 29: 850–860.

Kovalcikova, M., and Kovalcik, K. 1984. 'Learning ability and memory in cattle of different age.' In *Proceedings of the International Congress on Applied Ethology in Farm Animals*, (eds. Unshelm, J., Van Patten, G., and Zeeb, G.), pp. 65–69. Kiel.

Macha, J., and Olsarova, J. 1986. (Variability and heritabilities of grazing intensity in cattle). *Acta Universitatis Agriculturae – Brno*, 34, 313–320.

Mendoza-Ordones, G., Wilke, A., and Seeland, G. 1988. 'The importance of certain feeding traits of dairy calves as an aid to selection.' Berichte, *Humboldt Universitat zu Berlin*, 8, 62–67.

Mishra, R. R., Chauhan, R. S., and Gupta, S. C. 1975. 'Studies of dairy temperament of Karan Swiss cows.' *Indian Journal of Dairy Science*, 28, 85–88.

Mokhov, B. P. 1983. (Breeding of cattle for stereotyped behaviour). *Doklady Vsesoyuznoi Akademi Sel' skokkozyoistvennykh Nauk*, 9, 32–35.

New Zealand Dairy Board. 1961. *37th Farm Production Report, 1960–61*. Farm Production Division NZ Dairy Board, Wellington.

O'Bleness, G. V., Van Vleck, L. D., and Henderson, C. R. 1960. 'Heritabilities of some type appraisal tests and their genetic and phenotypic correlations with production.' *Journal of Dairy Science*, 43, 1490–1498.

Persson, E. 1978. (Analysis of test milking data). *Husdjur*, 11, 16.

Phillips, C. J. C., and Weiguo, L. 1991. 'Brightness discrimination abilities of calves relative to that of humans.' *Applied Animal Behaviour Science*, 31, 25–33.

Rottensten, K., and Touchberry, R. W. 1957. 'Observations on the degree of expression of oestrus in cattle.' *Journal of Dairy Science*, 40, 1457–1465.

Salcido, G. P., and Eugenio, L. 1979. (Estimation of heritability indices for body weight at weaning, one year and 550 days, pigmentation and temperature in a herd of Brahman cattle in Playa Vicente, Veracruz.) *Veterinaria*, 10, 194 (Abstr.).

Santha, T., Prieger, K., Keszthelyi, T., and Czako, J. 1988. (Genetic analysis of feeding behaviour of cows). *Allaltenyesztes-es-Takarmanyozas*, 37, 501–514.

Sato, S. 1981. Factors associated with temperament of beef cattle. *Japanese Journal of Zootechnical Science*, 52, 595–605.

Shrode, R. R., and Hammock, S. P. 1971. 'Chute behaviour of yearling beef cattle.' *Journal of Animal Science*, 33, 193 (Abstr.)

Stricklin, W. R. T., Graves, H. B., Wilson, L. L., and Singh, R. K. 1980. 'Social organisation among young beef cattle in confinement.' *Applied Animal Ethology*, 6, 211–219.

Warwick, V. D., Arave, C. W., and Mickelsen, C. M. 1977. 'Effects of group, individual and isolated rearing of calves on weight gain and behaviour.' *Journal of Dairy Science*, 50, 947–953.

Wickham, D. W. 1979. 'Genetic parameters and economic values of traits other than production for dairy cattle.' *Proceedings of the New Zealand Society of Animal Production*, 39, 180–193.

CHAPTER 3

PLAY

WHAT IS PLAY?

Play behaviour is difficult to define and even difficult to consider as only one sort of behaviour, with a common goal and motivation. In general parlance 'play' is often used to refer to actions performed for the amusement of the performer and other animals involved in the activity. This alludes to the difficulty in defining the *objectives* of play. In behavioural terms 'play' refers to activities with definable characteristics (Loizos, 1966), but most of these differ from other behaviours only in scale.

Components of play are exaggerated or repeated versions of other behaviours, particularly infrequently used ones such as fighting, fleeing and copulation that are used for survival. The sequence of the components of the behaviour may be reordered or incomplete and usually lacks the consummatory phase. Play is preceded and accompanied by signals that the behaviour *is* play, and typically playmates interchange roles frequently.

General manifestations in cattle are:

1. *Mock fleeing* Running, trotting, cantering and galloping, often with tail elevated.
2. *Mock aggression*
   - Bucking with both hind feet jerked up posteriorly and often to one side with an accompanied lateral twist of the hind quarters.
   - Kicking with one or both hind feet, often at moving objects. Also pawing the ground with front feet.
   - Head butting with playmate, head butting stockmen or movable objects, goring and head pushing movements.
   - Prancing and mock challenges, with head lowered or shaken

27

from side to side, often accompanied by snorting.
- Vocalisation, varying in type with the degree of excitement. Most vocalisations are normally of low amplitude and frequency (Kiley, 1972).
3. *Mock copulation* Mounting other playmates, inanimate objects and even stockmen, sometimes with pelvic thrusts. A large proportion of mounts are disorientated—head to head, head to side, intention mounts and solicitation. Mock copulation is not accompanied by penile erection or vaginal intromission.
4. *Environmental exploration* Investigation of novel objects in the environment, in particular to determine their reactivity—patterns of movement, noise, etc.

Some age effects are evident in cattle play. The first forms of play are usually solitary and, for obvious reasons, are usually mock fleeing such as running, gambolling and jumping. Calves may also be involved in play with adults, especially their mothers, at an early age. In older calves play is usually between calves of similar age and involves social play more frequently, particularly head pushing and mounting (Vitale *et al.*, 1986) (Plate 3.1).

Sex differences also occur. Male calves more often initiate and are the recipient of play than female calves, and they are more often the protagonists. Males also partake more in combative play. Examina-

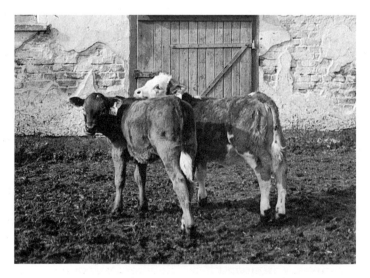

Plate 3.1   Older calves often indulge in social play.

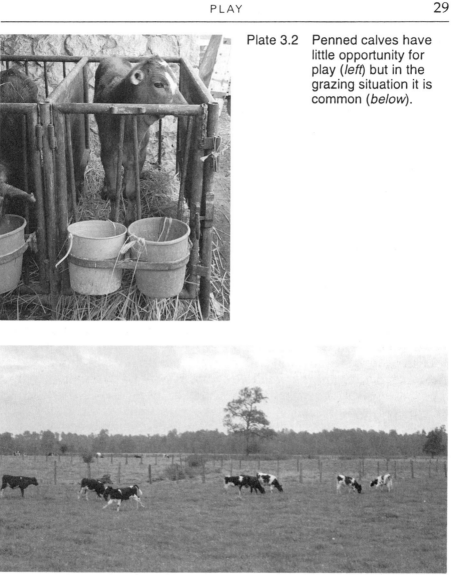

Plate 3.2 Penned calves have little opportunity for play (*left*) but in the grazing situation it is common (*below*).

tion of temporal variation shows that play activities are most common in mid morning and mid afternoon, and are rare at night. With housed cattle the incidence of play is directly correlated with light intensity in the house, and this could be related to the psychosomatic condition of the animal (Dannenmann *et al.*, 1985). Play behaviour is often thwarted in housed calves due to inadequate space, but is common in grazing calves (Plate 3.2).

FUNCTIONS OF PLAY

Play contains components of many behaviours but may arise from a single motivation. Because of its multicomponent nature, it is difficult to ascribe a single function to play.

Early theories of play function were sometimes negative, regarding it as useless, perhaps a vestigial behaviour from some period of evolution. Indeed it has even been cynically referred to as the 'wastepaper basket of imperfectly understood animal behaviour' (Loizos, 1966). We should, however, acknowledge that play itself is still poorly understood. For instance, it may be indistinguishable from stereotypic behaviour in some circumstances. These early ideas coincided temporally with the Victorian belief that 'children should be seen and not heard', thus denigrating play in both animals and man as a worthless activity. This belief was not without some logic, however, as play is normally restricted to well-fed animals and can be seen as their means of dispersing excess energy. Although some of this energy could be stored in mature animals as fat tissue, in the juvenile this is not common. In the absence of normal releasers other methods have to be found of dissipating the energy, and in this respect it *is* relevant that well-fed animals play more frequently than poorly fed ones (Brownlee, 1954).

This energy dissipation theory fails to acknowledge a biological value of play per se. That there must be such a value is suggested by the fact that animals demonstrate motivation for play (Hinde, 1970). However, play clearly has a lower priority than behaviours essential for body maintenance—feeding, drinking and sleeping. As a result highly productive dairy cattle, which spend up to two-thirds of their time in ingestive behaviour (grazing and ruminating) alone, play very little in comparison with calves that spend only one-tenth to one-quarter of their time in ingestive behaviour.

The widely supported motor training theory proposes that play serves to exercise muscles, often those associated with infrequently used survival functions such as flight, agonistic behaviour and reproduction. These muscle groups are then strengthened by vasodilation and the survival function enhanced. In support of this theory we find combat play more common in male than female calves, in preparation for the greater role that combat normally plays in the adult male. It is difficult, however, to explain 'intellectual' play, an animal playing with a light switch, for example, or the random, rather illogical nature of play if it is purely for exercise.

It is frequently proposed that play serves to increase and stimulate learning. This is certainly true of learning the features of the environment, and novel environments stimulate play. Animals also learn their position in the dominance hierarchy through play, which prevents damaging aggressive interactions later on. Again the rather irrational nature of play is hard to explain if this is the main aim. Play also helps juvenile cattle to learn behavioural patterns and responses and thus serves as practice for adult function. However, only limited improvement of play characteristics is usually seen from the time the calf first starts playing, which may be a few hours after birth. Also play is not confined to juveniles: adult cows, for example, can take delight in charging round a field when the stockman is attempting to collect them for milking.

In prey animals play may also serve to keep the young together through social facilitation. The sight of two calves playing frequently acts as the stimulus for a third to join in. Isolated calves are more at risk from predation. Play may also go one stage further by strengthening social bonds to increase the cohesion of the herd and act as a catalyst for social facilitation.

A possible function of play that is not frequently considered is the psychological reward. Acknowledging that animals need psychological stimulation used to be thought an affront to man's superiority. However, the frequency of play is broadly correlated with the degree of cerebralisation in animals. Animals with a high degree of cerebralisation, especially primates, also perform more intellectually challenging forms of play. The size of the brain in ungulates is relative to that of the body, larger than in rodents or insects but smaller than in the higher mammals (MacPhail, 1982).

Play is encouraged by novel stimuli and in particular by tasks which are just beyond the immediate intellectual capacity of the animal. Cattle appear, for example, to gain satisfaction from playing with a latch on a door until they can open it. A state of psychological and physical well-being is a requisite for play. Fine, sunny weather stimulates play and increased light perception has been associated with endorphin release in the brain (see Chapter 1). Sick animals do not play, but this may be because energy reserves are conserved to combat the disease. There is therefore convincing evidence that animals receive psychological rewards from some forms of play, but it is difficult to judge whether these rewards are the objective of play, as most physically useful tasks involve some psychological reward. In addition, performing intellectually challenging tasks could increase cognitive powers, which again could have survival value.

Play is therefore a multicomponent behaviour almost certainly with more than one objective. As such we may be wrong in ascribing one term to it, and thinking of it as one behaviour only. This, however, is a problem which probably only reductionist research into neuroendocrinal control will answer.

REFERENCES

Brownlee, A. 1954. 'Play in domestic cattle in Britain: an analysis of its nature.' *British Veterinary Journal*, 110, 48–68.

Dannenmann, K., Buchenauer, D., and Fliegner, H. 1985. 'The behaviour of calves under low levels of lighting.' *Applied Animal Behaviour Science*, 13, 243–258.

Hinde, R. A. 1970. *Animal Behaviour, a Synthesis of Ethology and Comparative Psychology*. McGraw-Hill, New York.

Kiley, M. 1972. 'The vocalisations of ungulates, their causation and function.' *Zeitschrift fur Tierpsychologie*, 31, 171–222.

Loizos, C. 1966. 'Play in mammals.' *Proceedings of the Symposium of the Zoological Society of London*, 18, 1–9.

MacPhail, E. 1982. *Brain and Intelligence in Vertebrates*. 433 pp. Oxford University Press, Oxford.

Vitale, A. F., Tenucci, M., Papiri, M., and Lovari, S. 1986. 'Social behaviour of the calves of semi-wild Maremma cattle, Bos primigenius taurus.' *Applied Animal Behaviour Science*, 126, 217–231.

CHAPTER 4

SOCIAL BEHAVIOUR

Animals are generally classified as solitary, aggregated or social. Social animals employ communicative behaviour that transcends sexual union, and aggregated animals maintain a lower inter-individual distance than equidistant spacing in the environment, but without communication other than sexual. Cattle are social animals in the fullest sense of the word, with complex communication channels and allelomimicry common to many behaviours.

In order to truly understand the social behaviour of domesticated cattle, the reasons for the cohesive forces that existed in non-domesticated cattle must be appreciated. These animals grazed in unisexual groups, and the size of the group was determined by the balance between the reduced risk of predation due to aggregating and the increased competition for scarce resources, particularly feed and a mate. Forming a herd reduced the risk of predation by leaving large areas of grazing land devoid of cattle and reducing the chance of a predator seeing the animals or picking up a trail. Predation was probably also reduced by the rapid flight of large numbers of animals in a random direction, thereby confusing the predator. The effectiveness of tasks such as surveillance would be increased in a herd, but under conditions of low pasture availability the inter-animal distance would have been increased to ensure effective coverage of the total area. Also the opportunity for members of a herd to learn survival tactics was increased through social facilitation.

In addition to these factors favouring herding in wild cattle, domesticated cattle have even shorter inter-animal distances than other grazing ungulates (Lewis, 1978), which is probably due to selection by man for ease of herding over thousands of years. Domestication has allowed man to control cattle for productive purposes. To obtain full control man must usually displace the top-ranking animal in the

33

dominance order. This is readily accomplished by most competent herdsmen with a herd of cows, but it is difficult, for example, in a herd of bulls, which are naturally more aggressive and stronger than cows. A herdsman may form a 'social pact' with bulls, and even top-ranking cows, whereby both tolerate each other's presence, but agree to minimise contact that could result in aggressive interaction. If regular close contact with bulls is unavoidable, strong expression of human dominance is required. For example, Fulani tribesmen are noted for their aggressive attitude to bulls from birth because the management system necessitates frequent close contact with all their cattle. Dominance of all the cattle by the tribesmen is a necessity, rather than a social pact, and this can only be achieved by aggressive control of the bulls from birth (Lott and Hart, 1977).

SOCIAL INTERACTIONS

Social interactions form the communicative medium for social information transfer. They are an initial part of environmental *exploration*, which is followed by *recognition* of environmental cues. Once position in society is established, regular *communication* is used to maintain status and assess environmental changes. Finally *bonding* occurs between the animal and the features of its environment.

Exploratory Behaviour

Exploration is the exhibition of investigatory behaviour to other animals (usually herdmates) or inanimate objects, and is maximised in yearling cattle (Figure 4.1) (Murphey *et al.*, 1981). In the immediate postnatal period exploration is directed primarily towards the dam and not to the environment, as adequate defensive behaviour has not yet been established, e.g. fleeing. Innate maternal behaviour by the cow causes her to lick the calf and eat the placenta. There then usually follows a refractory period, when cattle are fearful of novel stimuli, but it is not clear whether this still occurs if the neonate and dam are separated soon after birth, as in most dairy production systems. After exhibiting attraction to the dam, the calf will display attraction to its environment and peers. In general the more complex the environment, the more exploratory behaviour is displayed (Kenny and Tarrant, 1987). This period of exploration eventually declines but can be restarted if the animal moves to a new environment or is placed with a new group of cattle.

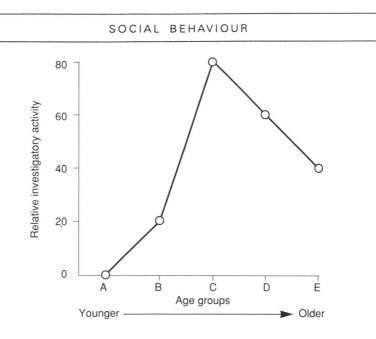

Figure 4.1   Relative investigatory behaviour in different classes of cattle.
A = preweaned calves; B = weaned calves; C = yearling heifers;
D = two-year-old heifers; E = adult milking cows. (Murphey et al., 1981)

Recognition

Recognition of herdmates allows social interactions to be conducted
without the need for repeated dominance establishment. It is mainly
achieved by vision, although sound is also important for maternal-
juvenile recognition. Olfactory confirmation takes place at close
quarters, but the visual and vocal cues provide the primary recognition responses and are additive in line with Seitz's (1940) law of
heterogeneous summation of stimuli (Soffie and Zayan, 1977). There is
a high degree of specificity, allowing recognition of the sight or sound
of herdsmen or an individual herdsman for example (Murphey and
Moura-Duarte, 1983). However, little is known about the scope of the
recognition memory of cattle. It has been suggested that cows can
recognise 50–70 herdmates (Fraser and Broom, 1990), and if this is true
it could explain why herds larger than this tend to be subdivided. A
cow is able to recognise her calf after only a few minutes of contact
after parturition. The exploratory licking by the cow reinforces the
bond and aids subsequent recognition by the addition of salivary
pheromones to the calf's coat (colour plate 2).

Communication

As prey animals, non-domesticated cattle would have been discouraged from excessive use of intra-special communication because it attracts the attention of predators. However, domestic cattle have lost some of these inhibitions, especially as adequate communication is of vital importance in an intensively managed gregarious species.

Visual communication

Visual signals, which are one of the commonest communication methods, are particularly used by cattle to indicate aggressive and reproductive state.

In the case of aggression, the signals confirm and reinforce the recognition or dominant position of participating animals. Threats are given which represent an intention to attack. In bulls this takes the form of lowering the head and inclining the horns to the opponent (colour plate 3), with intention charge actions such as pawing the ground. Other threat activities include neck and head rubbing on the ground (Plate 4.1), which is not visual communication but to mark the ground with salivary pheromones. These activities during the threat display indicate the intention to pursue and execute a direct physical and violent attack on the other animal. In cows the threat is less forceful and generally involves a head swing towards the opponent.

In both the male and female the tail is often elevated and may wag. The degree of elevation of the tail is related to postural tonus, and a highly elevated tail is generally associated with display behaviour. Submission is usually indicated by lowering the head and tail and turning away, as if to retreat. Actual retreat indicates a greater degree of submission. The objective of the submissive display is to indicate acceptance of the dominance of the opponent, by lowering/belittling parts or all of the body and suggesting retreat.

Reproductive display is similar in the bull to the threat display, but in the cow reproductive receptivity is indicated to bulls, other cows (to invite the formation of a sexually active group) and not least to man, by homosexual mounting and standing to be mounted. Some indication of appeasement is necessary and flehman is believed to fulfil this function as an antithesis to the threat display. The cow exhibiting the standing reflex is receptive, not necessarily the mounting cow.

The body elevation provided by homosexual mounting would have been particularly useful to cows grazing extensively in tall, open grassland, where the bulls would form a separate herd some distance

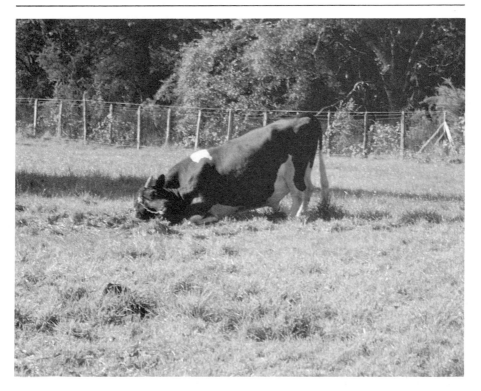

Plate 4.1   A neck and head rubbing display in a bull.

away (colour plate 4). Mounting cows, although not necessarily receptive, are usually approaching receptivity so their activity is not entirely reciprocal altruism, as they themselves may benefit from the presence of a fertile bull. In domesticated cattle, where the bull is normally removed from the herd, such homosexual mounting is of great benefit to the herdsman to indicate the right time to bring in a bull or to use artificial insemination.

Olfactory communication

Olfactory sensitivity is greater in cattle compared with man (see page 8), and it is therefore likely that it is relatively more important in social communication. The chemical messengers used for intra-special social communication and also for interspecial communication are called pheromones. They are secreted by interdigital, infraorbi-tal, inguinal, sebaceous and salivary glands and are particularly concentrated in the perineal region. They are also present in milk, urine and the other body secretions.

As described in Chapter 1 odours are received through both the nose and the vomeronasal organ in cattle. The vomeronosal organ characteristically receives them by the flehman facial expression in which the head and neck are extended upwards, the lips are curled back and air is sampled through a partially opened mouth. The vomeronasal organ is particularly involved in receiving pheromones that control aggressive behaviour and the oestrous cycle of cows. Bulls can detect a change in the pheromenal secretions of cows up to four days before the day of oestrus (French *et al.*, 1989). On the day of oestrus the main olfactory system of nasal detection is operative and flehman is not always used. The ability of bulls to predict oestrus in cows relates to their tendency in wild herds to 'guard' cows as oestrus approaches. In domestic herds where there is no competition between bulls this does not occur. To test for cows' odours bulls sample the urine of potential oestrous cows (colour plate 5) and mark the ground with pheromones by rubbing their head and neck on the ground. Homosexual cow behaviour is stimulated by sniffing and licking, particularly in the perineal regions (Plate 4.2). Other animals, such as dogs, cats and rats, can also detect the oestrous odours of cows, but they are not able to discriminate preoestrous odours from those produced at other stages in the cycle in the way that bulls can.

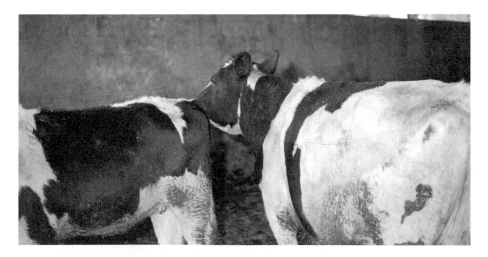

Plate 4.2   An oestrous cow sniffs the anovaginal area of another oestrous cow to detect the pheromones.

Tactile communication

Tactile communication is mainly used in aggressive encounters, allo-grooming and sexual behaviour.

Aggressive encounters   In aggression the main forms of tactile interaction are charging, head pushing, butting and occasionally kicking. Mounting can be said to have both aggressive and sexual functions (Klemm *et al.*, 1983). Charging is used primarily by bulls (Plate 4.3). Head pushing is characterised by locking of horns in horned breeds and by contact between foreheads. Heads are lowered to exert maximum force and a rigid stance is adopted (colour plate 6). Each animal attempts to overpower/outmanoeuvre its opponent and gain access to butt the vulnerable flank or udder area. Often the losing combatant will wheel around in an attempt to prevent access to the flank area (Plate 4.4). Violent butting at the end of the bout is usually avoided:

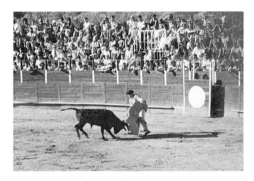

Plate 4.3   The charge by a bull.

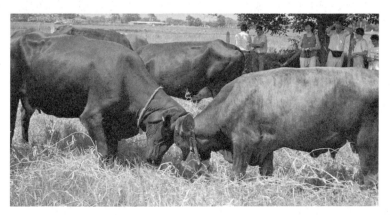

Plate 4.4   In head to head contact, cattle wheel around, each attempting to overcome the other by the strength of the pushing.

the purpose of the fight is to establish dominance and only the 'threat' of injury is used. This type of fighting is common in bulls and cows, whereas steers more commonly indulge in butting, aggressive riding and kicking (Hinch and Lynch, 1987).

Butting involves a characteristic upswing of the head usually to either the head or flanks of the other animals. The force of the movement varies from a mild push to a severe blow. Bunting is a similar action (the term is more often used to refer to the repeated pushing of the udder by a suckling calf to stimulate milk letdown).

Allogrooming Grooming is primarily a body care activity but it also has nutritional, communicative and psychological functions.

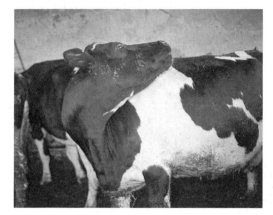

Plate 4.5   Self grooming by a dairy cow.

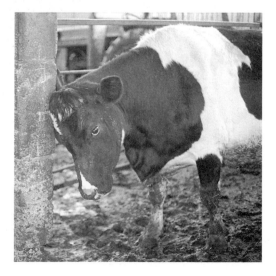

Plate 4.6   Head rubbing by a dairy cow against the corner of a wall.

Plate 4.7   Neck rubbing on the
             ground.

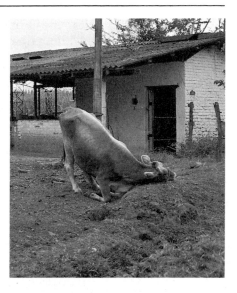

Plate 4.8   Allogrooming in two dairy
             cows.

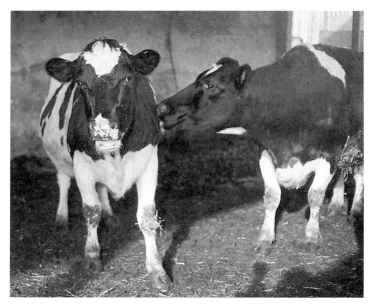

Self-grooming is characterised in cattle by licking activities (Plate 4.5),
but rubbing of the head (Plate 4.6) and neck (Plate 4.7) is also
common. Allogrooming (grooming others) is mainly licking the head
and neck regions of animals which are in a similar or slightly
subordinate position in the dominance order (Plate 4.8 and colour
plate 7). All animals are groomed but only about three-quarters of the

animals in a herd do the grooming (Sato, 1984). As preferred partners are often kin, allogrooming may thus function not only to maintain dominance position but also to reinforce family bonds and those between adult cattle. Fraser and Broom (1990) also attribute dopaminergic functions to allogrooming, suggesting that since the hormone prolactin is known to be associated with grooming and also dopaminergic activity, grooming may via prolactin cause opiate induction and self-narcotisation. The fact that allogrooming is increased in more intensive environments, where stereotypies are often performed for self-narcotisation, supports this hypothesis.

Sexual behaviour   Sexual behaviour is the third kind of tactile communication. Chin pressing on a cow's back by a bull or another cow tests for the rigid back stance and whether she will be receptive to mounting.

Allogrooming activity by members of a sexually active group (SAG) increases during oestrus, but in this instance the same attention is paid to the anovaginal area as to the head and neck. Immediately prior to coitus, direct stimulation of the vulval area by nudging by the bull is common.

Vocal communication

As gregarious grazing animals, cattle make more use of vocalisation for communication than solitary animals would, although it is used less than by true forest-dwelling species such as jungle fowl, where vocal communication is more effective than other communicative methods. The absence of predators in most farm situations probably explains why cattle, and in particular calves, are more vocal than other grazing ungulates. In the social context vocalisation is used for recognition and eliciting contact, as well as greetings, threats and fear display (Plate 4.9).

Although specific cattle calls cannot be identified and their range of vocalisation forms a continuum, certain types of call can be associated with different behaviours. For instance, as the animal becomes more excited the length, amplitude and pitch of the calls increase.

Cattle calls may be classified according to several characteristics (Kiley, 1972):

The Syllables   Five main syllables are used (best represented by m, en, en, h and uh), although these are not mutually exclusive. The 'm' syllable is produced with the mouth shut and the sound emitted through the nostrils. 'En' is produced with the mouth open, and most of the sound emitted from the mouth rather than the nose. The glottal

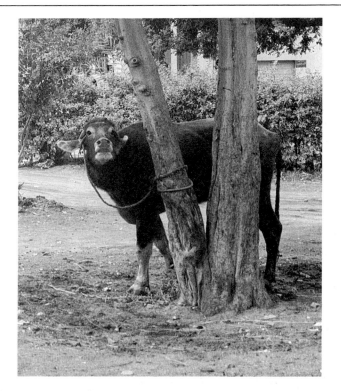

Plate 4.9 Open mouthed vocalisation in a
tethered buffalo.

lips may be tightened as the pitch increases. The 'en' sound is usually
a sudden increase in frequency and amplitude from the 'en' sound
and is the same phenomenon as overblowing a wind instrument.
The 'h' sound is produced with an open or closing mouth as the
diaphragm and lips relax after the 'en' sound. Finally the 'uh' sound
is produced during rapid inspiration.

These five syllables are combined into six major calls, again not
mutually exclusive: mm, men(h), (m)enh, menenh and two see-saw
calls, (m)(en)enh and menenhuh (Table 4.1).

Amplitude This is generally less for calls such as mm, where the
mouth is closed, and is greater for the en than en sound.

Pitch This is generally increased as amplitude increases. The fundamental tones are typically 50–1000 Hz but the overtones can reach

TABLE 4.1 Description of the characteristics of cattle calls.

			CALL			
	mm	*men(h)*	*(m)enh*	*menenh*†	*(m)(en)enh**	*menenhuh**
Duration (sec)	1–3	0.5–4.1	1.0–2.8	0.8–3.5	0.7–2.3	1.3–2.9
Repetition	Variable	up to 10X	Variable	up to 10X	1–20X	1–10X
Amplitude: *m*	low medium	low medium		medium	medium	medium
en		medium–high	high	medium–high	high	high
en		low–medium		high	medium	high
h			high	medium		high
uh						medium–high
Pitch *m*	50–125	50–125		75–100	75–125 rising	75–125 rising
(Hz) *en*		125–300	125–250	100–250	175–500 falling	250–750 falling
en				500–800		1000–1250
h				100 falling		
uh						
Tonality: *m*	high	medium–high	medium–high	medium–high	high	medium
en		medium–high		medium–high	medium	low–medium
en				medium–high	medium–high	low–high
h					high	low
uh		low	low	low	low	low–high

X = times
* see-saw calls
† may precede see-saw calls
(After Kiley, 1972)

4–8 kHz in the en syllable, which is near the hearing limit in man but within that for cattle (see page 6). In the loudest calls the pitch alternates between high and low in much the same way that human singers sustain a note by alternation of the pitch (vibrato). The pitch of a call also indicates social status in that the freedom to vocalise at a higher pitch is reserved for more dominant animals (Hall *et al.*, 1988).

Tonality   This is the musical quality of the sound as determined by the variation in frequency of the note. The fundamental tone is the lowest frequency sound, and there are also overtones which are multiples of the fundamental but less audible.

Length   Length refers to both the duration of each call and its frequency of repetition. Most calls are 1–3 seconds in length, this being restricted by the maximum duration of expiration. Cattle in a more excited state are more likely to repeat a call.

Message   The mm call indicates a mild level of excitement as when a familiar herdmate or herdsman approaches, during anticipation of a pleasurable event such as milking or feeding, or during courtship. It is also used by bulls guarding oestrous cows and for recognition purposes, since the long wavelength of the sound facilitates intra-aural localisation.

The men(h) call indicates a state of slightly increased excitement and is commonly referred to as a 'moo' or, in the old English, 'low'. It may be uttered in situations of mild frustration as when cattle are waiting for food, are isolated from the rest of the herd or are mildly fearful. It is the commonest of all cattle calls in most herd situations.

In the (m)enh call the degree of excitement and tension is heightened, such as when a cow has her calf removed, when cattle are very hungry and often by bulls during the threat display. The menenh call is an extension of this where the animal is in its greatest state of excitement and is often colloquially referred to as a 'holler' or 'roar'.

The two see-saw calls are primarily produced by bulls in an excited state and by the change in frequency they emphasise the excited state of the caller. They are also part of the dominance display and may inhibit other bulls from agonistic acts (Plate 4.10).

Bulls tend to vocalise more than cows and steers and are particularly vocal in spring and summer (Figures 4.2 and 4.3). Cows and calves in the wild vocalise more in winter, possibly because of the low availability of feed at this time. Calves normally use vocal communication primarily for contact maintenance. Calling by all cattle, especially bulls, is strongly socially facilitated.

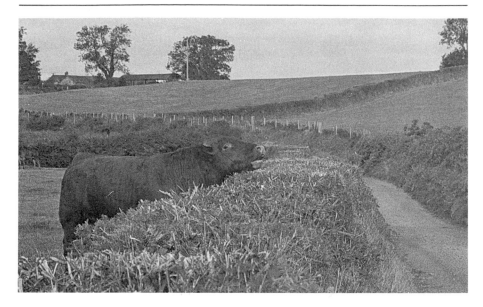

Plate 4.10   A bull indicates his attraction to cows the other side of a hedge by high amplitude, open-mouthed vocalisation.

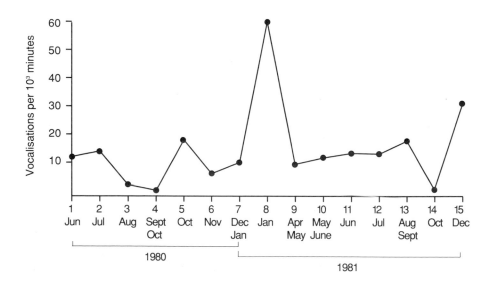

Figure 4.2   Cow vocalisations expressed as number of vocalisations per thousand minutes of observation time. (Hall et al., 1988)

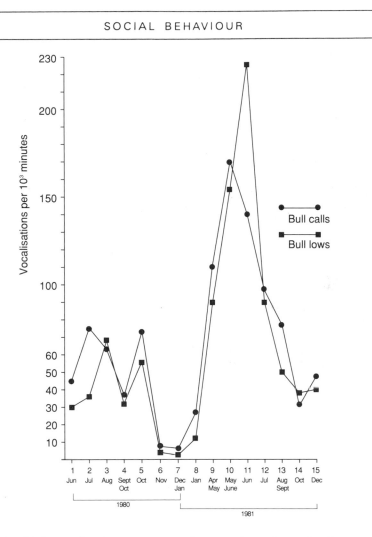

Figure 4.3   Bull vocalisations expressed as number of vocalisations per thousand minutes of observation time. (Hall *et al., 1988*)

Intra-special Bonding

Mother-filial bonding

In cattle it is the female parent, rather than the male, which normally becomes bonded to the offspring. This bonding initially develops soon after birth and, given the opportunity, will persist as a matriarchal family group (Reinhardt and Reinhardt, 1981). The initial bonding, which is termed imprinting, has the following characteristics. It develops during a 'sensitive' period, which for a precocious animal such as *Bos taurus* occurs in the immediate postnatal period. It is permanent and irreversible but its relative importance will depend on the strength of other imprinted bonds which the dam has. A cow with twins develops a weaker bond with each calf than a cow with a single calf, and this encourages the twins to form sibling bonds (Price *et al.*, 1986). Within a semi-wild herd of cows and calves the bond between dam and daughter will persist as the dominant social force (Reinhardt and Reinhardt, 1981), whereas the males disperse to form bachelor groups. Equal preference is generally given by the dam to her off-spring, regardless of their age and sex.

Multiparous cows form stronger bonds than primiparous cows through greater contact and contact-seeking behaviour, and they are more disturbed by separation (Price *et al.*, 1986). Primiparous cows show more abnormal maternal behaviour but are reported to spend longer suckling their calves than multiparous cows, perhaps because the milk flow rate is less. The creation of a strong maternal-filial bond is therefore a learnt characteristic, although much of the stimulation behaviour by the calf is innate. Intensively selected dairy breeds such as the Friesian show weak dam-filial bonding. They are more easily cross-fostered and removal of the calf for artificial rearing has little effect on its temperament, whereas in less developed breeds such as the Salers (Le Neindre, 1989 a, b) artificial rearing reduces the social adaptiveness of the calves. In all breeds, artificially rearing calves *in isolation* reduces their social adaptiveness compared with group-reared calves and results in them occupying lower positions in the dominance order in later life (Plate 4.11). Isolation rearing is often advocated to reduce between-calf contact and risk of disease spread at a time when the animals are very susceptible to infection. It stresses the calf, but this seems to condition the animal to accept stress in adulthood and may encourage a good relationship between the stock-man and his cattle rather than strong bonding between cattle.

Thus it can be seen that cattle are socially adaptable, and in the absence of a preferred social partner they strengthen the bonds with other partners. For the young calf the dam is the preferred social partner, followed by kin, other peers and lastly other species such as humans.

Imprinting tends to occur within species, but is not confined to certain classes of individuals (Thorpe, 1963). However the bond is created at a time when the calf is naturally drawn to the dam by suckling motivation and the chances of other bonds being created during the period of primary socialisation are small. The bond is preserved by grooming during and after suckling, but other forms of communication like vocalisation must be important, since calves that

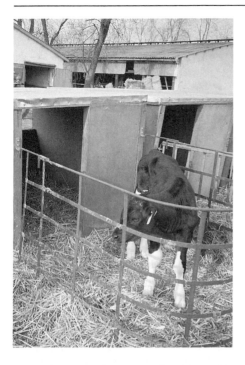

Plate 4.11 Calves reared in partial isolation (*left*) cannot form sibling bonds as they do when reared in an open field (*below*).

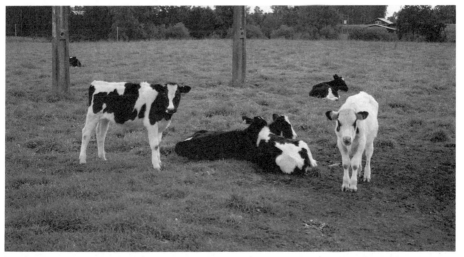

are muzzled to prevent suckling and grooming still develop a bond with their dams. The bond, and in particular suckling, maintains the post-partum anoestrus in the cows for about 8 weeks to prevent early rebreeding.

The benefits of a strong mother-filial bond are many, particularly in wild cattle. For the dam the need to perpetuate the family line is paramount—the 'selfish gene' (Dawkins, 1976). For the calf the initial reward is in the form of protection: the afterbirth and other residues are consumed by the dam to minimise the risk of predation, and nutrition is provided in the form of milk. Early licking of the perineal region stimulates the functioning of the gastrointestinal tract and excretion (Kovalcik *et al.*, 1980). Later the calves learn dietary and other habits from their dams (Provenza and Balph, 1987) and acquire a stable position in the herd structure.

Peer bonding
The first evidence of peer relationships usually comes in the first or second week of life of the calf. The dam may leave her calf in a 'crèche' of other calves whilst she grazes nearby. Often she remains within sight of the calves. If she does not, as may occur in extensive grazing conditions, another cow may keep watch over the nursery. Crèches are more often formed under extensive grazing conditions, where the cows need to leave the calves to cover the area effectively (Plate 4.12). Typically the calves spend 2–5 hours/day in the crèche and leave it when they need to begin grazing, after about 10–15 weeks. Under intensive grazing conditions calves usually stay with their dams or may play with peers whilst their dams graze.

Juvenile-juvenile bonds are more likely to occur between siblings, because sibling calves are brought into frequent contact with each other through their mother. The bonds are maintained through play and grazing associations, not by allogrooming, as is the case with

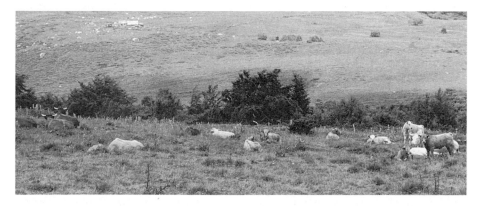

Plate 4.12   Peer bonding in extensively grazed cattle. Cows associate with each other on the left and calves with each other on the right.

adult cattle. The formation of the bonds is irrespective of the sex of the calves, but male-male bonds are likely to be broken earlier than female-female. Sex differences which relate to adult function appear in their play. Males indulge more in mounting play which enables them to learn correct orientation and timing of mounting. This enhances their performance, as adult males and bulls that have not had this practice are not so reproductively capable (Silver and Price, 1986). Homosexual mounting may persist in groups of intensively housed adult bulls, and some subordinate bulls may be excessively ridden as a form of aggression by the dominant bulls. Usually, however, it is the bulls with more masculine conformation that are ridden more and show more aggressive behaviour (Jezierski et al., 1989).

In adult cows peer bonds are preserved by allogrooming and grazing and less by play. Allogrooming (see page 40) is generally unidirectional, i.e. only one partner grooms, whereas most grazing partnerships are bidirectional, i.e. both animals prefer to graze with each other (Reinhardt and Reinhardt, 1981). Only about 20% of partnerships are common to both grazing and grooming associations, so different partners are usually chosen for the two activities. Not all adult cows, however, develop associations, as some prefer to remain solitary.

Inter-special Bonding

The intensification of agriculture during the last half century has led to increased emphasis on single species farming, without the complexities of mixed farming. During this period less emphasis has been placed on efficient natural resources utilisation, which is often greater in mixed farming systems, and more emphasis has been on labour efficiency, which often necessitates single species farming if high output is to be achieved. With the achievement of greater self-sufficiency in many agricultural commodities in developed nations in the 1980s, there was more interest in mixed farming systems, partly because of the increase in pasture utilisation and the reduced need for unsustainable parasite control measures. Cattle and sheep were traditionally recognised as good grazing partners (Plate 4.13), and cattle and goats have similar advantages of pasture utilisation complementarity. Normally the two species graze separately in species groups, but there is considerable overlap in areas utilised. This preserves intra-specific social cohesion and minimises inter-specific conflict. In competitive situations horses dominate cattle, which in turn dominate sheep (Arnold, 1984).

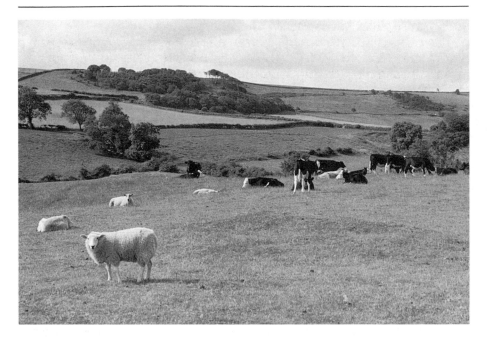

Plate 4.13   Cattle and sheep are good grazing partners, especially as
sheep will graze the areas around cattle faeces that cattle
reject and vice versa.

In extensive grazing conditions protection of the smaller ruminants
from predators can be achieved by bonding them to the cattle. In the
Americas the coyote and the puma still cause an appreciable risk of
predation of both adult and juvenile sheep and goats, despite the
increasing loss of the predators' natural habitat. This may prevent
farmers keeping sheep or goats, particularly near forests or in silvo-
pastoral systems. Domesticated dogs or horse patrols can be used for
protection but are not very effective at night. Systems of protection have been developed of bonding the small ruminants to cattle,
usually heifers. Normally this can be achieved by penning young
sheep or goats with the cattle for about 60 days, although a longer
period is necessary if the cattle show aggressive tendencies to the
young animals. When the bond is formed inter-specific distance is
reduced and during an attack protection is achieved by the sheep
positioning themselves amongst the cattle (Anderson *et al.*, 1988),
whereas non-bonded sheep would move away from the cattle.

The bond between cattle and man

Cattle, being social animals, seek alternative bonding if their matriarchal groups are disrupted. Man may assume the role of most dominant animal, mother, offspring substitute or leader. Acting responsibly as the boss 'animal' brings stability to the herd, and there is evidence that cattle respond best to a person who is confident and consistent in handling them (Seabrook, 1984). The cattle also respond to regular communication with the stockperson, particularly during periods of stress such as calving. This communication may be in the form of touching the animals, petting, stroking or scratching, particularly around the head area. This mimics grooming by conspecifics and maintains the bond between man and cattle. Communication may also be verbal and visual, with good stock people regularly talking to and looking at the cattle in their charge. The importance of a stockperson's olfactory signals to cattle is not fully understood, but there is evidence that this plays an important role and may even enable cattle to know a person's mood before any other communication has taken place.

Much of the effective communication between the stockperson and cattle should be to confirm the relationship between them. Firm handling to assume dominant status combined with the caring role of the matriarchal substitute is necessary if the cattle are to be contented. There is increasing evidence that contented, unstressed cattle grow faster and produce more milk (Seabrook, 1984). Unfortunately many modern production systems are designed for minimal labour input and the importance of the stockperson's role in the herd is not recognised (colour plate 8). Abnormal behaviour problems in the herd may increase as a result, and a farmer's time and money may be wasted devising physical methods to overcome these problems without recognising the psychological needs of the cattle for adequate social bonding. Stereotyped oral behaviours in calves and mounting behaviour in bulls or castrates are examples of these abnormal behaviours.

SOCIAL ORGANISATION

Social Hierarchies

In semi-wild or wild cattle, herd social organisation takes the form of matriarchal groups, consisting of mother and offspring, and bachelor groups of bulls. In domesticated cattle, however, these natural groupings are replaced by groups of cows and growing cattle, usually divided into similar age and single sex groups after about 6 months of age. Bulls kept for reproduction may be solitarily confined for much of their life, or they may be run with a herd of cows or rotated between herds. These changes in the social structure from the natural groupings and the intensive husbandry methods used increase social tension. In the case of bulls the stress caused by close confinement may make them difficult to manage safely or without danger to the stockperson, and castration is often performed to improve their temperament. In all intensively managed stock a strict hierarchy develops to determine priority of access to resources. The existence of a hierarchy reduces aggression by eliminating the need for repeated agonistic encounters to determine priority, thus ensuring that scarce resources are rapidly and easily given to the strongest and fittest animals.

The hierarchy is not the same for all resources because some individuals attribute more importance to certain resources and will fight harder to gain access to them. Separate hierarchies can be demonstrated for access to feed, space, sexual partners and milking, although several of these show close correlation. The order of greatest concern in intensive husbandry situations is usually the hierarchy for space priority, which is usually referred to as the dominance order.

Dominance order

This hierarchy has been variously referred to as a hook, bunt, peck, rank, aggressive or competitive order, social rank or dominance status. It indicates spatial priority because it is measured by observing agonistic interactions between cattle when space availability is reduced, e.g. in a passageway or other confined area. Space allocation, and more particularly the preservation of personal space, is at the heart of social organisation. Other hierarchies, e.g. order of entry into the milking parlour, are less keenly contested.

As the dominance order becomes established in a herd, the aggression becomes ritualised, and little more than a nod of the head may be needed to confirm status by the dominant animal and a slight avoidance movement by the subordinate animal. Allogrooming confirms dominant status (and to a lesser extent the other hierarchies), and acceptance of a conspecific's superiority is at least partly controlled by pheromones. Animals close in the dominance order need to confirm status more regularly, and changes in order may occur in 25% of the herd annually. Older members of the herd with an established position initiate less aggression, because experience in the herd conveys social advantage and may frustrate the rank ambitions of younger members. Younger members must constantly challenge older members to elevate their position in the hierarchy.

The prime determinants of rank are therefore age, weight and size. Although weight and size are correlated with age, the social skills necessary for gaining a high rank need to be learnt. This usually occurs partly as juveniles during play, and animals reared in spatial isolation are usually dominated by animals reared in groups (Broom and Leaver, 1978). Most studies have, therefore, found age to be the prime determinant of rank (e.g. O'Connell *et al.*, 1989).

In addition to experience and physical ability, a third factor, emotionality or fear, determines dominance and varies in importance in different individuals. Of the three factors it is likely that physical ability is most important in a highly competitive situation, as animals learn to overcome their fear to obtain priority of access, and the benefits of experience are less of an advantage if agonistic encounters are frequent and young members can rapidly learn the art of social elevation. Under these circumstances young members of the herd

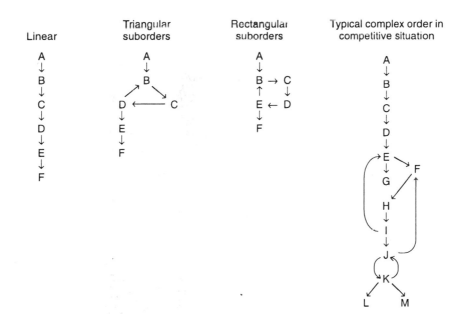

Figure 4.4   Dominance orders, with triangular and rectangular suborders. (Beilharz and Mylrea, 1963 a and b)

may therefore increase their status factor faster than in less competitive situations. In more competitive situations complex relationships are formed and the order may develop from linearity to include triangular and even more complex relationships (Figure 4.4). Physiological status will affect an animal's position in the dominance order. Oestrus elevates it to enable cows to obtain access to a partner and pregnancy reduces it to limit the risk of damaging aggressive encounters (Beilharz and Mylrea, 1963 a,b).

The variation in aggressive tendencies between individuals has long been the subject of debate, not least as we try to explain our own self-destructive inclinations. Lorenz (1966) argues in favour of an endogenous supply of aggression, which, when supplemented with environmental triggers, necessitates release through agonistic acts (Figure 4.5). The relative absence of aggression in wild/semi-

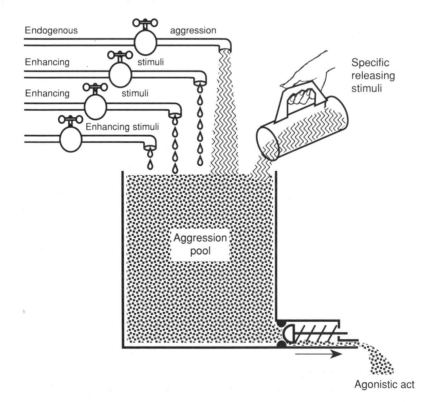

Figure 4.5   Lorenz's hydraulic model of aggression. (Lorenz, 1981)

wild cattle herds with adequate resources suggests that in cattle, at least, environmental stimuli are more important than endogenous stimuli. Individual variation in aggressive tendencies in competitive situations may relate to, first, variation in pain perception, second, the individual's determination to maintain access to resources and, third, position in the dominance order. High-ranking individuals show more aggression than low-ranking ones (Collis, 1976), but this may arise from the need to maintain status rather than any genetic disposition.

The dominance or spatial hierarchy is particularly important in intensive husbandry because there is little opportunity for escape for low-ranking individuals. They have to move about more to avoid high-ranking individuals (Arave et al., 1974) and this creates stress. Spatial priority also relates to access to lying areas, in particular cubicles. Preferred cubicles—those in the centre of a line or those with enclosed fronts that offer more privacy—will be occupied by high-ranking cows at preferred times. Low-ranking cows are left to occupy them at less preferred times or to occupy less preferred cubicles. Generally at least 0.9 cubicles/cow are considered adequate to avoid competition for cubicles.

Feeding order
Rank determined by competitive feeding behaviour is closely correlated with rank determined by spatial encounters (Rutter et al., 1987). However, some compensation for having a low priority of access is possible in the case of feed restriction. When feed is spatially distributed so that high-ranking individuals cannot prevent low-ranking ones from feeding, there is little need for a feeding order. This generally occurs with grazed feed, even if the availability is less than that required to give an ad libitum intake. In the case of conserved forages offered at a feeding barrier, dominant animals will usually eat at preferred times and subordinates at less preferred times, unless there is space for all to eat at once. An allowance of 15 cm manger space per animal is adequate for beef and dairy cattle to obtain ad libitum intake.

If forage availability is restricted, the rate of eating of conserved feeds will be increased to a certain extent, but not enough to allow the dominant cows to eat a great deal more than their fair share (colour plate 9). Position in a feed priority order may become especially important if concentrate feeds are offered in restricted amounts to a group of cattle. Cattle usually prefer the concentrates to the forage, and considerable aggression may result as dominant cows attempt to get more than their fair share. Individual feeders have therefore been devised which ration the concentrates to a programmable allowance every few hours, or for lactating cows they may be placed in the milking parlour to allow intakes of up to approximately 5 kg per milking. Artificial milk replacer can be similarly rationed mechanically for calves.

Milking order

Milking order, or the order of presentation of the cows for milking, is only weakly related to the dominance order. There is some tendency for more dominant cows to enter the milking parlour earlier but it is more likely to be the higher yielding cows. The reward that entering the parlour offers depends on the frequency of milking, the milk yield of the cow and the provision of concentrates. If cows are milked just twice a day and the intervals are uneven, e.g. 16 hours overnight, 8 hours during the day, then high-yielding cows will suffer from high udder pressure before morning milking, and will experience a greater reward than low-yielding cows. Cows with subclinical or clinical mastitis are more reluctant to enter the parlour, as milking may cause discomfort (Rathore, 1982). If concentrates are offered in the parlour, cows with priority of access for food will tend to enter early. At a given stage of lactation high-yielding cows are likely to be more hungry than low-yielding ones because of their more rapid removal of fermentation end products. However, early lactation cows may be less hungry than late lactation cows because the gut is involuted.

Maintaining the same order of entry into the milking parlour does not seem to be of major or lasting importance to the cows. It is not related to the peer associations and can be readily rearranged through training. Although some rearrangement of order is readily tolerated, cows do prefer to be milked at approximately the same time each day. In a block calving herd the order is not clearly defined when the cows are in early lactation but becomes more ordered in mid to late lactation.

Sexual partner priority

In many modern husbandry systems the function of natural reproduction is superseded by artificial insemination using specially selected male genes, or even by embryo transfer using selected male and female genes. In less intensive systems bulls are used but the male:female ratio is much lower than would naturally be the case (colour plate 10). It is only in large, extensively managed herds, usually kept for beef production, that several bulls may be run together and there is a possibility of priority to sexual partners by dominant bulls. In such circumstances dominance, and in particular age, is important in determining which bulls serve most of the cows. In one herd with four bulls aged two to ten years, over two-thirds of the cows were served by the oldest bull (Blockey, 1978). This dominancy was achieved by the top male refusing other males access to the sexually active group of females. Only when four or more cows were in heat simultaneously were other bulls able to serve the cows. If there were fewer cows, attempts to copulate by the subordinate bulls were interrupted. The aggregation of receptive females into a sexually active group helps the dominant male to maximise the inheritance of his genes and is therefore an evolutionarily useful behaviour. As reproductive priority is so closely linked to genetic inheritance, it is to be expected that strong dominance effects will be present in the fight to gain access to receptive females. The genes therefore demand that the most dominant bull serves to his capacity before other bulls are given opportunities. Unfortunately the most dominant bull is not necessarily the most fertile and the herd reproductive rate can be reduced.

Spatial Distribution

Cattle arc aggregated into non-random patterns, both when housed and at pasture. For economic reasons, stocking densities on farms are normally greater in the cattle house than at pasture; however, milking cattle kept in sheltered woodland choose to operate at greater inter-individual distances than in the open range (Dudzinski et al., 1982), suggesting that cattle under cover prefer a lower stocking rate than in the open. This dichotomy can lead to social tension in the cattle house as it has been seen that the maintenance of personal space is one of the main status symbols for cattle. The personal space is the envelope or 'bubble' around each individual that it attempts to keep free from interference by other animals. When this space is breached, the animal will attempt to flee from the intruder. Studies of both housed and grazing situations show that cattle expend a great deal of effort in maintaining the correct inter-individual distances (colour plate 11), and this is something which we as humans may find difficult to grasp. It is only on those rare occasions that we move into a very different stocking density that we may feel uncomfortable, e.g. when a person from the country enters a crowded underground station, or a city dweller becomes agoraphobic in uninhabited countryside.

The distance from an animal's head to the edge of the 'bubble' is known as the flight distance (colour plate 12). Because the animal's senses are concentrated towards the reception of signals from the

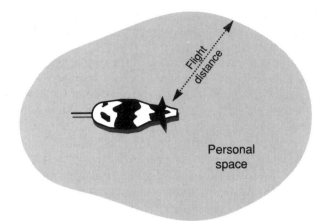

Figure 4.6 Personal space and flight distance.

front, the flight distance is greater in front of than behind the animal (Figure 4.6).

Flight distance is determined by the environment, the type of cattle and their position in the dominance order. In intensive environments the flight distance is by necessity reduced compared with, for example, an open range. Beef cattle have greater flight distance than dairy cattle, even in the same environment, demonstrating that short flight distance has been selected for during the domestic evolution of dairy cows.

Animals higher in the dominance order have greater flight distance and normally intersperse themselves throughout the herd to avoid contact with each other (Beilharz and Mylrea, 1963 a,b). This means that less dominant cattle continually have to move around to avoid contact with the dominant cattle. In a cubicle house they often seek respite in less preferred cubicles such as at the end of rows, but in an open yard or small paddock where there is no escape for subordinate cattle the incidence of agonistic encounters is increased (Kondo *et al.*, 1989).

Forced movement of cattle initially creates an order unrelated to dominance, because the dominant cattle are interspersed throughout the herd. However, low-dominance cattle gradually move to the front and the most dominant animals stay in the middle. The dominant cattle may be said to lead the herd by 'pushing' rather than 'pulling'. They are reluctant to be right at the back of the herd because their attitude relative to the humans driving the group is often more fearful than medium- and low-dominance cattle. Less dominant cattle have been found to be more likely to escape from the herd, as they are relatively less afraid of humans than the more dominant cattle.

In free movement of cattle in the grazing situation a small benefit might be expected from leading the herd, because the leaders get first access to the pasture. This may not be very great, however, as some researchers have measured no relationship between dominance and position in the grazing herd. Others have said that the medium-dominant cattle lead the herd, most-dominant are in the middle and least-dominant follow. Not all cattle are closely associated with the herd. Some low-dominance cattle graze more independently, and presumably this reclusiveness demonstrates an antipathy to or a fear of agonistic interactions.

Most cattle herds graze in a pear-shaped formation, which may be simplified into a parallel formation in small herds or where there is considerable benefit from having first access to the sward, e.g. in strip grazing. Normal inter-animal distance under good grazing conditions when the size of the paddock is not limiting is about 10 m (Kondo *et al.*, 1989). The presence of flies, which are attracted to the secretions from the lacrimal and sebaceous glands (Plate 4.14),

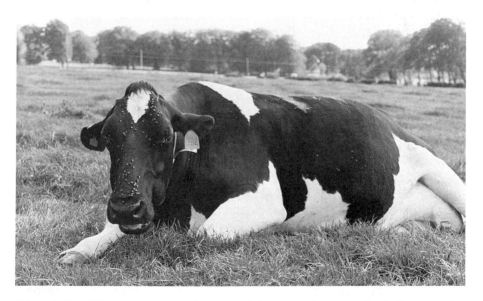

Plate 4.14 Flies are attracted to glandular secretions, particularly around the face in cattle.

causes the cattle to reduce the inter-animal distance. With heavy fly infestation, cattle will rest from grazing by standing with their heads together (Plate 4.15) or will seek elevated ground where wind may reduce the number of flies. Tail swishing and head movements, including ear flapping, reduce the infestation. Excessive heat may also disrupt the grazing process. Shade-seeking is not always a synchronised behaviour, and may be performed in turn by members of the herd (colour plate 13).

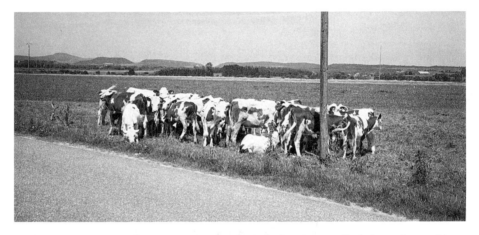

Plate 4.15   Young cattle bunch together during heavy fly infestation, with their tails swishing to provide a deterrent.

Although the size of the enclosure for cattle is often dictated by economic considerations, the shape of the enclosure can be manipulated to allow for the social behaviour needs of the cattle. With housed cattle the perimeter : area ratio should be maximised because cattle use the perimeter ground more than any other. This ratio is greatest for a rectangle and increases as the length to breadth ratio increases; it is least for a circle. In the grazing context, overuse of the grazing by the perimeter fence may necessitate a minimisation of this ratio to graze the whole area of the field evenly.

Bulls develop individualistic behaviour as they mature, and will pace up and down perimeter fences. They will also overgraze corners. In rangeland conditions these behaviours do not develop until the bulls are three to four years old, but in intensive grazing they occur much earlier. During the time when bulls develop their territoriality they show much agonistic activity, particularly head to head encounters. If space allows they create special areas, often choosing elevated ground, for display and threat behaviour, and subordinate bulls are often excessively mounted or ridden after agonistic encounters. Again, if space allows, the bulls once mature will remain in their own territory to minimise agonistic encounters. The most dominant bulls have the largest territories. In these circumstances grazing loses its synchronised character and bulls are not orientated in the same direction during grazing (Kilgour and Campin, 1973).

Herd Size and Space Allowance

As herd size increases individual members have difficulty remembering the social status of other members. The frequency of agonistic encounters then increases, at least in cattle where a dominance order has been established. In young calves where no dominance order has been formed, group size has no effect on the frequency of agonistic encounter (Kondo et al., 1989). Cattle decrease their inter-animal distance in response to increased group size, especially calves, who have not learnt their position in the dominance order and the need to refrain from invading other animals' personal space (Plate 4.16). The detrimental effects of a large group size can be overcome, where space allowance is adequate, by the formation of subherds or smaller groups within a population. This frequently occurs in beef cattle on rangeland, where herds typically break up into groups of 10–12 animals. When cattle are brought together for the first time there is initially aggression, to determine dominance, followed by aggregation. In the small groups agonistic encounters are initially more frequent but quickly these produce repeatable results and the encounters can then be ritualised and become less frequent (Kondo et al., 1989). Small groups show more rapid aggregation, whereas large groups take longer to become stable.

An increase in space available to the herd results in an increase in the inter-animal distance for both calves and adult cattle. In adult cattle the need to retain cohesiveness of the group at high space allowances is evident as they have a maximum inter-animal distance of 10–12 m above a space allowance of 360 m^2 per animal (Kondo et al., 1989). In all cattle the frequency of agonistic encounter decreases as space allowance increases. This may reduce stress but it does not always increase the growth rate of beef cattle or milk yield of dairy cattle.

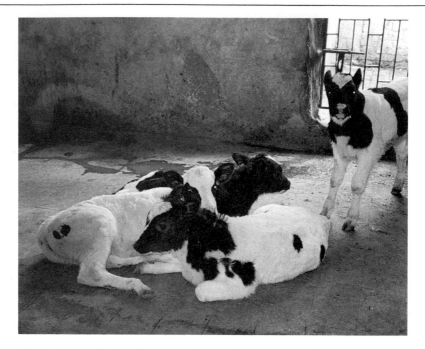

Plate 4.16 Calves have not learnt the concept of personal
space, and do not refrain from close proximity.

Space Perception

An animal's perception of space is undoubtedly influenced by many
environmental and physiological factors, and it is much more complex than, for example, a simple volume measurement. The quality of
space available, and therefore the space requirement, are affected
by building factors such as lighting; the number, design and size
of cubicles; flooring characteristics; the width of feeding and other
passageways; the waste disposal system and the number and type of
feeding and drinking stations (Potter and Broom, 1987).

Animal factors which influence space requirements include the
physiological state of the animal, its sex, the presence of horns and
the breed of cattle. Physiological state is important, for example,
when periparturient cows distance themselves from the rest of the
herd. Sex is more important in adult than juvenile cattle, and even
the body form (male or female type conformation) influences the
behaviour and social space requirements. Bulls with more masculine body characteristics are more aggressive and more dominant,
but surprisingly they initiate fewer and receive more mountings

(Jezierski *et al.*, 1989). This may occur because bulls of the more dominant masculine type pose a constant threat to subordinate, more feminine type bulls, who attempt to meet this challenge by mounting their rivals.

Breed effects are clearly discernible in the social behaviour of cattle and probably relate to the length and type of domestication influence as well as the physical environment. Hill breeds normally dominate lowland breeds, even if they are smaller: e.g. Aberdeen Angus dominate but are smaller than Herefords (Stricklin, 1983). They also tend to have a greater flight distance and less readily accept artificial management practices, such as bucket rearing (le Neindre and Sourd, 1984). Crossbred cattle dominate and are more aggressive than purebred cattle, which may be one reason for the popularity of purebred cattle for dairy herds, despite the production advantages for the crossbred.

Animal and environmental effects on space perception such as these must be included in the design of accommodation for any cattle farming system. Ideally the needs of all the cattle should be accounted for, but frequently, extremes of body size, temperament, age, etc, as for example in regard to cubicle size, do not receive special allowances.

Isolation

Isolation is generally not a natural state for such gregarious animals as cattle, but there *are* occasions when they prefer to be solitary. A cow that is about to calve normally seeks an isolated place so that she can give birth undisturbed and, more importantly, the calf will be drawn to the correct dam without the risk of mismothering (Edwards, 1983). Mature bulls also seek territorial isolation from other bulls, although they may remain within sight of one another. Subordinate and sick cows often graze away from the rest of the herd, presumably to avoid agonistic encounters with more dominant cows. Sexually active cows, either with a bull or other cows, usually isolate themselves from the rest of the herd. These are the situations in which cattle seek at least partial isolation from the rest of the herd, but modern husbandry methods often impose isolation at quite different times.

The most contentious period of isolation in modern cattle farming is that of the newborn calf. Calves are usually separated from their dam at about 24 hours post-partum and offered artificial milk replacer for five to seven weeks in individual pens. This is done to prevent cross-infection at a time when the calves' natural immunity is not well developed.

The imprinting or primary socialisation drive appears not to be fully satiated by the initial 24 hour contact between cow and calf, since longer contact increases the bond between the two, and hence the stress of separation. This isolation delays or eliminates the normal refractory period after primary socialisation and the calves attempt to create substitute bonding partners to replace the severed imprinting bond. Group-reared calves quickly form associations amongst themselves but delay the formation of a dominance order unless resources are restricted.

Individually reared calves have at most visual contact with a small number of calves and perhaps tactile contact with nearest neighbours (see Plate 4.11). Stronger bonds may be created with stockmen and therefore, particularly if the same stockmen are responsible for the adult cattle, this will strengthen the relationship to the stockman in adult life. Signs of behavioural deprivation, however, are common and the calves' behaviour is affected for life. In their pens they often display redirected behaviours, particularly those related to the absence of suckling contact with the dam such as sucking the pen, buckets or 'kissing' the nearest neighbour. That this is not solely caused by the deprivation of suckling is demonstrated by the absence of these behaviours in group-reared calves fed artificial milk replacer. Locomotion is by necessity limited and individually reared calves vocalise more by higher frequency 'baaocks' (see (m)enh on page 44) than the normal 'moos', indicating greater stress. When they are eventually put into groups they are socially maladapted, and this loss of experience is never compensated for. These calves are denied a crucial period of play which restricts their social development. In comparison with calves that are given cattle contact from birth, they are less skilled, particularly in social contact situations, and they tend to be less dominant. They are also less successful in agonistic interactions and are less skilled sexually, with more disorientated mounting behaviour (Silver and Price, 1986). These differences are maintained into adulthood.

The experience of stress at an early age is probably of benefit to calves if the environment during adulthood is going to be stressful (Creel and Albright, 1989). There is an argument that juveniles should be conditioned to adult stresses, and there is good endocrinal evidence that this will facilitate stress habituation in adulthood (Creel and Albright, loc. cit.).

Other instances of enforced isolation in modern cattle farming systems include the separation of sick dairy cows and dairy bulls from the rest of the herd. Individual tethering of dairy cows is also still common in many countries, particularly in hot countries where feed must be cut and fed to the animals under shade and/or countries where labour is sufficiently available for this purpose. In developed countries loose housing, where the cows are given the free range of the building, is practised increasingly because of high labour costs. Frequent human contact can at least partially substitute for the intra-specific bonds, and hence the traditional system of keeping dairy cows in individual stalls can function satisfactorily with adequate labour inputs.

The isolation of sick cattle and dairy bulls causes stress, as evidenced by the frequent vocalisations of such animals (an attempt to increase social contact by vocal means where visual contact is prevented), increased aggression to stockmen and stereotypic behaviour. It could be argued that in the wild these animals are at least partially isolated from the herd, but what causes the stress is the completeness of the isolation in the case of the dairy bull housed in a bull pen, as well as the suddenness of it in the case of a sick cow that is withdrawn from the herd. In the prevailing atmosphere of increased awareness of animal rights, regular social contact is probably one such 'right' that a social species such as cattle should be afforded.

Mixing Groups

When cattle groups are mixed, a new dominance relationship is created, usually within 24–72 hours, depending on the degree of change in the group. Minor changes result in an approximate doubling in aggression activity for about 24 hours, longer if dominant cattle are introduced to a stable group. In bulls and to a lesser extent steers the increased aggression is accompanied by an increase in homosexual mounting and chinresting. This has given rise to the suggestion that mounting behaviour is stimulated by aggressive motivation rather than sexual attraction, but it would also be expected that the novel partners presented in a new group would stimulate sexual motivation. After regrouping there is a gradual transition from physical encounters to psychological (threat/avoidance) ones (Kondo and Hurnick, 1987).

Regrouping commonly occurs towards the end of an animal's life when it is mixed with other cattle in a truck and perhaps again in a market and/or abattoir. Creation of a new dominance order may be prevented, either by spatial restriction in a truck or lack of time in the market or abattoir. An increase in stress is evident during this period and has an adverse effect on meat quality due to a lowering of glycogen levels in the muscle tissue. This occurs during fighting and mounting activity in bulls preslaughter, so it is probably best to slaughter as soon as possible after the animals arrive at the abattoir.

In dairy cows changes in group structure may sometimes cause sufficient disruption to reduce feed intake and hence milk production. Normally this is not the case and the operation of feeding systems where cattle are grouped and regrouped during the lactation period into different yield levels will not usually adversely affect milk production (Konggaard *et al.*, 1982). The maximum recorded reduction in milk production after regrouping is of 4% for 5 days (Jezierski and Podluzny, 1984).

TEMPERAMENT

Temperament may be described as a major parameter in the personality or mood of cattle in relation to their reaction to man. It is genetically unrelated to position within the dominance orders, which primarily refer to priority of access to resources between members of the herd. In fact the within-breed heritability (h^2) of temperament is low, between 0–0.15 (see Chapter 2), and there are strong environmental (management) effects on temperament, primarily previous handling experience—its frequency, the animal's age when it was handled (temperament develops at an early age) and the degree of pain or unpleasant feeling associated with the handling. However, there are clear genetic differences between breeds, particularly between *Bos indicus* and *Bos taurus* cattle.

Despite the apparently low heritability, many breeding indices now include an assessment of temperament. In dairying more docile cows are known to give higher milk yields, and in *Bos indicus* cattle they also are quicker to letdown their milk. *Bos taurus* cattle tend to be more docile anyway in the milking parlour than *Bos indicus* and this is a result of extensive breeding for this characteristic. In beef and dairy cattle a consideration of an animal's temperament is particularly important in minimising the stress reaction, and higher productivity in both beef and dairy systems has been found in placid cattle in stressful situations. Stress-susceptible or 'fearful' cattle find it difficult to relax in a large, highly stocked, loose housing environment and they actually milk better in tie stalls (Devyatkina, 1986). The basic problem with stress in modern cattle housing is not the individual occasion but repeated stress reactions which elevate blood cortisol concentrations and reduce the growth rate of beef cattle, the milk production of dairy cattle and the reproductive rate (via gonadotrophin inhibition) of beef and dairy cows. The temperament of a dairy bull is also important for the ease of handling and safety of the stockman. Work rates are reduced if stockmen find themselves chasing cattle or having to give excessive encouragement to animals to move.

An animal's temperament should be measured in relation to its 'fearfulness', not 'aggressiveness'. Fearfulness will more often be expressed in an attempt to flee, or in excessive kinetic activity, rather than aggression towards the handler, which is more likely to reflect position in the dominance order. Fearfulness is best recorded in the parlour for dairy cows or in the crush for beef cattle. To a certain extent this represents a reaction to confinement as well as to the presence of humans. The optimal situation in which to measure fearfulness is when cattle are accustomed to the confinement, and it is the response to the approach or tactile stimulus from the handler which is recorded.

A number of scoring techniques have been devised, some of which include descriptions such as 'placid', 'docile', 'nervous', 'lively' (e.g. Nayak and Mishra, 1984), and they correlate well with the more objective measures of heart rate and breathing rate.

Normally cattle improve their temperament and become less fearful with age (Roy and Nagpaul, 1986), as they actually experience little unpleasantness with most handling experiences and habituate to them. It is likely that handling experiences during calfhood to a large extent formulate the animal's personality, as bad handling during this critical period will render an animal nervous and hypersensitive to stress.

The benefits of conditioning calves to a certain amount of stress by isolation have been detailed on page 66. It can be argued that to some extent mood is relative, and that an idyllic calfhood followed by transfer to stressful intensive husbandry conditions will be more detrimental to the animal's welfare than some stress conditioning during early life followed by more benign conditions in later life.

Cattle also respond to human temperament and this will affect their response to handling. Seabrook and Bartle (1992) have identified three major types of interactions between animals and stockmen: hand and arm (tactile) interaction, vocal interaction and holistic empathetic interaction (smell and other senses). Interactions may be either pleasant (patting the back, stroking, etc) or aversive (hitting etc) and performed with a varying degree of confidence by the stockman. However, even 'unpleasant' handling may be perceived as beneficial if it relieves the boredom of a sterile environment. Regular 'pleasurable' touching of the cows by the stockman has been clearly shown to be associated with high milk production (Seabrook, 1984). However, a certain amount of respect or fear for the stockman is necessary to enable him to move cattle with ease and discourages the cattle from attempting to force interactions with the human.

Some behaviour differences between high- and low-yielding dairy cows suggest that yield can be affected by the animal's attitude to the stockman (Table 4.2). Stockman attributes that are associated with high-yielding herds are shown in Table 4.3. In particular it is important for stockmen to be able to assess an animal's temperament, so that they can predict its behavioural reactions to handling, milking, etc and modify their own behaviour accordingly.

TABLE 4.2 The variation in behaviour of dairy cows in high- and low-yielding units.

| | | Dairy unit results | |
Behaviour		Higher yielding	Lower yielding
Mean entry time to parlour	(sec./cow)	9.9	16.1
Field flight distance	(metres)	0.5	2.5
Approaches to observer	(no./min)	10.2	3.0
Dunging in the parlour	(no./hour)	3.0	18.2

(After Seabrook, 1984)

TABLE 4.3 Developing interaction: factors associated with the development of good empathetic stockmanship.

FACTOR	ACTION
Operant conditioning	— reward FAVOURABLE behaviour of animal — use of food and other positive stimuli as a distraction for negative interaction
Physical contact	— stroking and patting — scratching animal's head
Social identification	— use of voice and social gestures
Stability	— consistent action — confident action
Handling	— non-aggressive behaviour

(After Seabrook, 1984)

REFERENCES

Anderson, D. M., Hulet, C. V., Shupe, W., Smith, J. N., *et al.* 1988. 'Response of bonded and non-bonded sheep to the approach of a trained border collie.' *Applied Animal Behaviour Science*, 21, 251–257.

Arave, C. W., Albright, J. L., and Sinclair, C. L. 1974. 'Behaviour milk yield and leucocytes of dairy cows in reduced space and isolation.' *Journal of Dairy Science*, 59, 974–985.

Arnold, G. W. 1984. 'Spatial relationships between sheep, cattle and horse groups grazing together.' *Applied Animal Behaviour Science*, 13, 7–17.

Beilharz, R. G., and Mylrea, P. J. 1963a. 'Social position and behaviour of dairy heifers in yards.' *Animal Behaviour*, 11, 522–528.

Beilharz, R. G., and Mylrea, P. J. 1963b. 'Social position and movement orders of dairy heifers.' *Animal Behaviour*, 11, 529–533.

Blockey, M. A. 1978. 'Serving capacity and social dominance of bulls in relation to fertility.' *Proceedings of the First World Congress of Ethology and Applied Zootechnology*, Madrid, pp. 523–530.

Broom, D. M., and Leaver, J. D. 1978. 'The effects of group-housing or partial isolation on later social behaviour of calves.' *Animal Behaviour*, 26, 1255–1263.

Collis, K. A. 1976. 'An investigation of factors related to the dominance order of a herd of dairy cows of similar age and breed.' *Applied Animal Ethology*, 2, 167–173.

Creel, S. R., and Albright, J. L. 1988. 'The effects of neonatal social isolation on the behaviour and endocrine function of Holstein calves.' *Applied Animal Behaviour Science*, 21, 293–306.

Dawkins, R. 1976. *The Selfish Gene*. Oxford University Press, Oxford.

Devyatkina, G. S. 1986. 'Selection of cows for stress resistance.' *Zhivotnovodsto*, 9, 40–42.

Dudzinski, M. L., Muller, W. J., Low, W. A., and Schuh, H. J. 1982. 'Relationship between dispersion behaviour of free-ranging cattle and forage conditions.' *Applied Animal Ethology*, 8, 225–241.

Edwards, S. A. 1983. 'The behaviour of dairy cows and their newborn calves in individual or group housing.' *Applied Animal Ethology*, 10, 191–198.

Fraser, A. F., and Broom, D. M. 1990. *Farm Animal Behaviour and Welfare*. 3rd ed. 437 pp. Baillière Tindall, London.

French, J. M., Moore, G. F., Perry, G. C., and Long, S. E. 1989. 'Behavioural predictors of oestrus in domestic cattle.' *Animal Behaviour*, 38, 913–919.

Hall, S. S., Vince, M. A., Walser, E. S., and Garson, P. J. 1988. 'Vocalisations of the Chillingham cattle.' *Behaviour*, 104, 78–104.

Hinch, G. N., and Lynch, J. J. 1987. 'A note on the effect of castration on the ease of movement and handling of young cattle in yards.' *Animal Production*, 45, 317–320.

Jezierski, T. A., and Podluzny, M. 1984. 'A quantitive analysis of social behaviour of different crossbreeds of dairy cattle in loose housing and its relationship to productivity.' *Applied Animal Behaviour Science*, 13, 31–40.

Jezierski, T. A., Koziorowski, M., Goszczynski, J. and Sieradzka, I. 1989. 'Homosexual and social behaviours of young bulls of different geno- and phenotypes and plasma concentrations of some hormones.' *Applied Animal Behaviour Science*, 24, 101–113.

Kenny, F. J., and Tarrant, P. V. 1987. 'The reaction of young bulls to short-haul road transport.' *Applied Animal Behaviour Science*, 17, 209–227.

Kiley, M. 1972. 'The vocalisations of ungulates, their causation and function.' *Zuchtungskunde Tierpsychologie*, 31, 171–222.

Kilgour, R. and Campin, D. N. 1973. The behaviour of entire bulls of different ages at pasture. *Proceedings of the New Zealand Society of Animal Production*, 33. 125–133.

Klemm, W. R., Sherry, C. J., Schoke, L. M., and Sis, R. F. 1983. 'Homosexual behaviour in feedlot steers: an aggression hypothesis.' *Applied Animal Ethology*, 11, 187–195.

Kondo, S., and Hurnick, J. F. 1987. 'Progress of social stabilisation in dairy cows after grouping.' *Canadian Journal of Animal Science*, 67, 1167 (Abstr).

Kondo, S., Sekine, J., Okubo, M., and Adahida, Y. 1989. 'The effect of group size and space allowance on the agonistic and spacing behaviour of cattle.' *Applied Animal Behaviour Science*, 24, 127–135.

Konggaard, S. P., Krohn, C. C., and Agergaad, E. 1982. 'Investigations concerning feed intake and social behaviour among group fed cows under loose housing conditions. VI Effects of different grouping criteria in dairy cows.' *Beretning Jra Statens Husdyrbrugsforsog* No. 553, 35 pp.

Kovalcik, K., Kovalcikova, M., and Brestensky, V. 1980. 'Comparison of the behaviour of newborn calves housed with the dam and in the calf-house.' *Applied Animal Ethology*, 6, 377–380.

Lewis, J. G. 1978. 'Game domestication for animal production in Kenya: shade behaviour and factors affecting the herding of eload, oryx, buffalo and zebin cattle.' *Journal of Agricultural Science, Cambridge*, 90, 587–595.

Lorenz, K. L. 1966. *On Aggression*. Methuen, London.

Lott, D. F., and Hart, B. L. 1977. 'Aggressive domination of cattle by Fulani herdsmen and its relation to aggression in Fulani culture and personality.' *Ethos*, 5, 174–186.

Murphey, R. M., Moura-Duarte, F. A., Coelho-Novoes, W., and Torres-Penedo, M. C. 1981. 'Age group differences in bovine investigatory behaviour.' *Developmental Psychobiology*, 14, 117–125.

Murphey, R. M., and Moura-Duarte, F. A. 1983. 'Calf control by voice command in a Brazilian dairy.' *Applied Animal Ethology*, 11, 7–18.

Le Neindre, P. 1989a. 'Influence of cattle rearing conditions and breed on social relationships of mother and young.' *Applied Animal Behaviour Science*, 23, 117–127.

Le Neindre, P. 1989b. 'Influence of rearing conditions and breed on social behaviour and activity of cattle in novel environments. *Applied Animal Behaviour Science*, 23, 129–140.

Le Neindre, P., and Sourd, C., 1984. 'Influence of rearing conditions on subsequent social behaviour of Friesian and Salers heifers from birth to six months of age.' *Applied Animal Behaviour Science*, 12, 43–52.

Nyak, S., and Misha, M. 1984. 'Dairy temperament of Red Sindhi, crossbred cows and Murrah buffaloes in relation to their milking ability and composition.' *Indian Journal of Dairy Science*, 37, 20–23.

O'Connell, J., Giller, P. J., and Meaney, W. 1989. 'A comparison of dairy cattle behavioural patterns at pasture and during confinement.' *Irish Journal of Agricultural Research*, 28, 65–72.

Potter, M. J., and Broom, D. M. 1987. 'The behaviour and welfare of cows in relation to cubicle house design.' In *Cattle Housing Systems, Lameness and Behaviour* (ed. Wierenga, H. K., and Peterse, D. J.), pp. 129–147. Martinus Nijhoff Publishers for CEC, Boston/Den Haag.

Price, E. O., Martinez, C. L., and Coe, B. L. 1985. 'The effects of twinning on mother-offspring behaviour in range beef cattle.' *Applied Animal Behaviour Science*, 13, 309–320.

Price, E. O., Smith, V. M., Thos, J., and Anderson, G. B. 1986. 'The effects of twinning and maternal experience on maternal-filial social relationships in confined beef cattle.' *Applied Animal Behaviour Science*, 15, 137–146.

Provenza, F. D., and Balph, D. F. 1987. 'Diet learning by domestic ruminants: Theory, evidence and practical implications.' *Applied Animal Behaviour Science*, 18, 211–232.

Rathore, A. K. 1982. 'Order of cows' entry at milking and its relationships with milk yield and consistency of the order.' *Applied Animal Ethology*, 8, 45–52.

Reinhardt, V., and Reinhardt, A. 1981. 'Cohesive relationships in a cattle herd (Bos indicus).' *Behaviour*, 77, 121–151.

Roy, P. K., and Nagpaul, P. K. 1986. 'The influence of genetic and non-genetic factors on temperament and milking parameters in dairy animals.' *Indian Journal of Animal Production and Management*, 2, 11–15.

Rutter, S. M., Jackson, D. A., Johnson, C. L., and Forbes, J. M. 1987. 'Automatically recorded competitive feeding behaviour as a measure of social dominance in dairy cows.' *Applied Animal Behaviour Science*, 17, 41–50.

Sato, S. 1984. 'Social licking pattern and its relationships to social dominance and liveweight gain in weaned calves.' *Applied Animal Behaviour Science*, 12, 25–32.

Seabrook, M. F. 1984. 'The psychological interaction between the stockman and his animals and its influence on performance of pigs and dairy cows.' *Veterinary Record*, 115, 84–87.

Seabrook, M. F., and Bartle, N. C. 1992. 'Human factors influencing the production and welfare of farm animals.' In *Farm Animals and the Environment*. (ed. Phillips, C. J. C., and Piggins, D.). Commonwealth Agricultural Bureaux, Slough.

Seotz, A. 1940. 'Die Paarbildung bei einigen Cichliden.' *Zucktungskunde Tierpsychologie*, 4, 40–84.

Silver, G. V., and Price, E. O. 1986. 'Effects of individual vs. group rearing on the sexual behaviour of prepuberal beef bulls: Mount orientation and sexual responsiveness.' *Applied Animal Behaviour Science*, 15, 287–294.

Soffie, M., and Zayan, R. 1977. 'Responsiveness to social releasers in cattle: 1. A study of the differential and additive effects of visual and sound stimatic, with special reference to the law of heterogenous summation.' *Behavioural Processes*, 2. 75–97.

Stricklin, W. R. 1983. 'Matrilinear social dominance and spatial relationships among Angus and Hereford cows.' *Journal of Animal Science*, 57, 1397–1405.

Thorpe, W. H. 1963. *Learning and Instinct in Animals*. 2nd ed. 1963. Methuen, London.

CHAPTER 5

NUTRITIONAL BEHAVIOUR

In this chapter all the activities concerned with obtaining nutrients for cattle maintenance and productivity are considered. These are primarily feeding, drinking, rumination and elimination.

Cattle evolved primarily as grazing animals, that is they harvest feeds, usually still growing, from the strata of plant life near the soil. By derivation 'grazing' refers to the harvesting of grasses in the field, but it may also apply to the harvesting of other plants or parts of plants—legumes, maize stover, etc. (colour plate 14). Cattle will also feed from shrubs and trees (browsing), although their mouthparts are not well designed for this. Grazing by cattle usually entails mass harvesting of low-level plant material with little selectivity compared, for example, with sheep. Cattle will consume grass heads on tall stems individually, but this is not their main method of feed harvesting; rather it is an energetically expensive way of obtaining some palatable feed items.

INGESTION

Feeding Mechanisms

Cattle feed and drink using their lips, teeth and tongue. During grazing all three are used to secure the feed in the mouth before ripping it from the sward. When cattle eat loose feed, i.e. not connected to the soil, the tongue is used to a greater extent to manipulate a particle into the buccal cavity. More free-flowing materials like liquids or powders, are sucked into the open mouth by expanding the lungs.

Feeds are masticated or chewed by compression and severance between the upper and lower molars alternating on either side of the jaw (colour plate 15). The lower jaw is moved upwards and inwards to contact the upper jaw on one side, followed by a similar action to achieve contact on the other side. Through this process and with the addition of saliva, which lubricates the food as well as having digestive functions, a bolus of the more fibrous material is prepared, with most of the cell solutes released.

Following chewing, this food bolus is manipulated into the pharynx by the tongue and contact with the pharynx triggers peristalsis, or contraction of the oesophagus behind the bolus, to deliver it into the rumen. After this swallowing process a new portion of food is obtained and the cycle recommences.

Foraging Strategy

Cattle evolved, along with other ruminants, with a unique anti-predator, digestion-enhancing foraging strategy. They consumed primarily coarse grasses which need large amounts of chewing or mastication before they can be digested. To minimise the predation risk they evolved a strategy of consuming the grasses as rapidly as possible, followed by mastication later in relative safety when they lay down, mostly at night. Boluses of feed are regurgitated during this mastication process (rumination) by reverse peristalsis.

The forage selection policies adopted by cattle must provide for the optimum nutrient intake. Nutrient requirements vary with the physiological state of the animal (e.g. pregnancy, body fatness), its genetic potential for high productivity and the need to provide milk for offspring. Cattle are motivated to feed by hunger, which is alleviated by a feeling of satisfaction or satiation. Hunger is not, however, a broad-spectrum motivational force. Specific hungers (euphagias) exist to maintain the intake of the major nutrients (energy, protein and sodium at least), but the range is limited by the perceptive powers of the cattle (Figure 5.1). For most cattle the major limiting nutrient is energy, even though they have a well-developed buffering system in the form of body fat stores. Energy intake is governed not just by feeding behaviour constraints, but also gut and digestive capacities.

Exactly how cattle acquire the necessary knowledge to achieve this nutrient selectivity remains unclear. Some believe they have acquired innate wisdom (evidenced by euphagias) to select the optimum diet. However, we can be sure that they do **learn** some elements of selectivity, probably by operant conditioning and by allelomimicry. For example, avoidance of toxic plants such as rag-wort is learnt not inherited. Cattle that have grown up with small

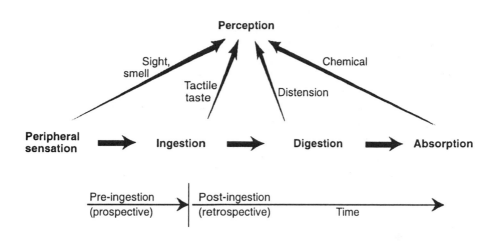

Figure 5.1   Flow diagram of the factors contributing to food perception (Illius and Gordon, 1990)

amounts of ragwort in a field learn of its mild toxic effect when eaten in small amounts and subsequently avoid it. However, if cattle are suddenly introduced to a field with a lot of ragwort and little alternative forage, and they have not experienced it before, they will eat large quantities with often lethal consequences. Learning evidently has an important part to play in dietary selection, but there are inherited elements too. That the grazing process itself is learnt is not in doubt. At 8 weeks of age calves graze at only 14 bites/minute but at 18 weeks this has increased to 50 bites/minute, a rate similar to that seen in adult cows (Hancock, 1953).

The manifestations of dietary selection are specific responses to feed characteristics—gustatory, olfactory and tactile. Some people believe that this is purely a hedonic response (hedyphagia) (see review by Provenza and Balph, 1990) but this ignores the fact that these hedonic responses almost certainly evolved in response to euphagias. However, although animals can be credited with a considerable degree of euphagia, this belief can be taken too far. There is, for example, the need for cattle to regularly sample the available forages to determine optimum forage intake (Illius and Gordon, 1990). Memory may therefore be limited. Even given a nutritionally optimum diet, it is likely that cattle would prefer variation in feed supply, and one long-standing technique of achieving very high intakes, and consequently milk yields, is to offer a wide choice of feeds to cattle. This was ably demonstrated in the 1940s at the Royal Agricultural College when Professor R. Boutflour achieved yields that are remarkable even by today's standards by offering a large range of feeds at regular intervals to cows. But for the difficulties of managing such a system, it would probably be popular today. This gives us clear evidence that some feed selection is hedyphagic rather than euphagic. Finally we must remember that we as humans do not always allow euphagia to influence our dietary selection, and hedonic responses often rule the day. In fact food manufacturers play on our hedonic drive by creating foods with unnaturally high sugar, fat and even salt concentrations, which we find difficult to refuse. In the same way it is possible to exceed the euphagic capabilities of cattle and, for example, increase the intake of forage by increasing its sodium content over and above requirements (Chiy and Phillips, 1991). However, some euphagia definitely exists and feeds with excessive sweetness or salt contents do have a reduced palatability (Chiy and Phillips, 1992).

Another force that controls foraging strategy apart from nutrient (primarily energy) intake optimisation is foraging cost minimisation. Up to a certain point—probably when cattle take about 50,000 bites over about 12 hours per day—there is only a small advantage to the animal in minimising foraging time as the energy costs of grazing are low in relation to total energy intake. However, as intake increases or availability of feed decreases, the opportunity cost of grazing becomes significant. In other words, foraging time begins to infringe on other highly desirable activities, e.g. resting. Metz (1984) has shown that, under certain circumstances, cattle prefer to maintain their full lying time rather than feeding time, when they do not have sufficient time for both activities.

An overriding concern of all grazing cattle is to satisfy their motivation for gregariousness, i.e. to stay close together, whilst feeding. Other behaviours, such as parturition, can be accomplished alone but grazing is a very social activity. Cattle develop preferred grazing partners (Reinhardt and Reinhardt, 1981) and adopt a common direction and interanimal distance during grazing (colour plate 11). The influence of this social facilitation process is clearly demonstrated when cattle are offered supplementary feed (Table 5.1). Cattle offered supplements reduce their grazing time, and when they are grazed with unsupplemented cattle the grazing times of the latter are reduced as well.

TABLE 5.1 The effects of social facilitation on the grazing response of cattle to a supplement of 3.6 kg oats per day.

	Grazing separately		Grazing together	
	Unsupplemented	Supplemented	Unsupplemented	Supplemented
Grazing time (h/day)	8.4	6.5	7.7	6.4

(Bailey *et al.*, 1974)

The Grazing Process

Cattle graze herbage by collecting it into the mouth and compressing it against the upper palate with the tongue and lower incisors. The herbage is then severed from the plants by jerking the head upwards. This is repeated several times a minute, typically 30–70, and the animal moves its head from side to side as it walks (Plate 5.1).

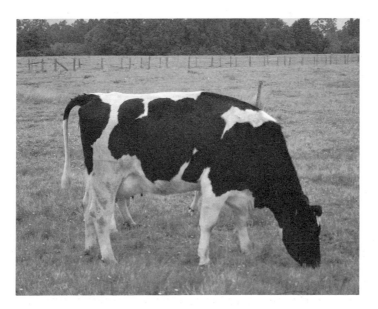

Plate 5.1   Dairy cows normally take 30–40,000 bites of grazed grass every day.

Associated with the grazing bites are occasional chewing bites or manipulative movements of the tongue or lips to manoeuvre the herbage in the mouth. These are more common when the herbage is long and fibrous. They are much less common in grazing cattle than in cattle eating conserved food, or in grazing sheep.

Cattle generally prefer to graze tall, dense and dark-green pastures. Some selectivity occurs even in the most uniform pastures. Herbage height largely determines the bite size or mass and a tall sward gives the greatest ease of prehension and therefore minimum foraging time. However, cattle do not exclusively graze tall swards and leave short areas untouched. When offering cattle a choice of 3 or 6 cm grass swards, James (1992) found that cattle only spent just over one-half of their grazing time on the tall sward.

Within any pasture there are also tall areas of herbage close to faecal deposits that are not grazed . The rejection around each faecal deposit will be greater in undergrazed swards because the cattle have the choice of other, clean areas to graze. Herbage around dung deposits is rejected initially because of the smell of the faeces and later because of its maturity. Typically it is lighter and browner than 'grazed' green herbage, and this indicates to the cattle that it has a low nutritive value. Darker green pastures are also usually preferred because this indicates a higher nitrogen content, and dense pastures because they give a greater bite weight. Cattle may be thought of as extracting a cylinder from the sward by the biting process, and if the herbage density is high this cylinder has a greater weight of herbage in it because of the large herbage weight per unit volume.

Although cattle are not as selective as sheep, their grazing action usually allows them to select a greater proportion of leaf material than the sward contains as a whole, thereby increasing the digestibility of their diet (Figure 5.2). This is primarily because of vertical selectivity: they graze the upper strata of the sward (i.e. above the pseudostems, normally about 2 cm above the soil surface), and this layer contains more leaf material.

Little is yet known about how cattle determine the height above ground level at which to defoliate the sward. They may balance a high leaf:pseudostem ratio (which would maximise nutrient content of the herbage) with achieving an adequate total intake. The extent to which they do this to optimise nutrient intake is as yet uncertain. According to the optimal foraging theory, the composition and volume of the plant eaten and the energetic cost of grazing and possibly digestion are believed to be optimised by the animal to supply its nutrient requirements at least cost in grazing time. The ease of severance of the bites may also influence grazing height.

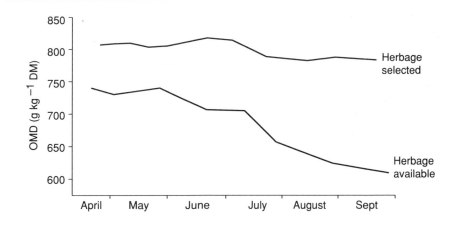

Figure 5.2 The organic matter digestibility (OMD) of herbage selected and of the available herbage. (Le Du et al., 1981)

There is horizontal selectivity against, for example, the herbage around dung deposits or herbage with hairy or waxy leaves. The opportunity for horizontal selectivity is limited by the mouthparts of cattle. Because of their uncleft upper lips and their broad dental arcade, cattle cannot manipulate individual plant items to the same degree as sheep and goats.

The sweeping side-to-side grazing action of each individual animal combines with the cohesive grazing action of a herd of cattle to result in a sward that is all, or nearly all, defoliated to a common height, with the exception of areas around dung deposits. In contrast, sheep select individual tillers and sever them much closer to the ground, providing a less frequent but more severe defoliation. This has its effect on the sward itself: because of the reduced frequency of defoliation, more tillers escape grazing altogether and become rejected due to their maturity, especially if the stocking rate of the sheep is too low. With cattle this only usually occurs in herbage around dung deposits, and even this is limited if the stocking rate is high. This ability of cattle to keep a pasture relatively free from mature herbage has led to their commonly being kept to 'clean up old pasture' on predominantly sheep farms. There are even greater advantages if cattle and sheep actually graze together, as the sheep do not show an aversion to cattle dung deposits and will prevent herbage near it from becoming mature and wasted.

In a mechanistic model of the cattle grazing process the feed intake can be determined from the grazing time multiplied by rate of intake (Figure 5.3). The latter can be further subdivided into bite mass and rate of biting, and the bite mass determined from the herbage density and bite size or volume. Bite volume is the product of bite area and bite depth. Bite area is a function of palate breadth and the distance between the palate and the tongue when the mouth touches the sward. Bite depth is the main factor regulating the other behavioural factors, and it is largely determined by sward height. Hence on a 10 cm lush spring pasture, intake rate is about 25–30 g DM/min, whereas a 5 cm autumn pasture will only be eaten at 15–20 g DM/min.

The compensation for reduced bite depth by other behavioural factors, principally grazing time and biting rate, may mean that herbage intake is not reduced by short swards. The ability of cattle to compensate depends on the severity of the bite depth reduction and the animal's intake requirements (Figure 5.4). If the intake requirements are high, the ability of the cattle to compensate is limited.

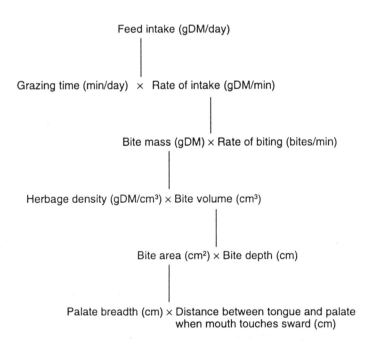

Feed intake (gDM/day)

Grazing time (min/day) × Rate of intake (gDM/min)

Bite mass (gDM) × Rate of biting (bites/min)

Herbage density (gDM/cm³) × Bite volume (cm³)

Bite area (cm²) × Bite depth (cm)

Palate breadth (cm) × Distance between tongue and palate when mouth touches sward (cm)

Figure 5.3   Mechanistic model of the grazing intake of cattle.

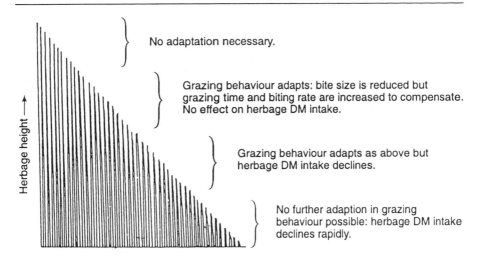

Figure 5.4   Effect of declining herbage height on grazing behaviour and herbage DM intake.

Maximum grazing times and biting rates normally occur at about 10–12 hours/day and 65–70 bites/minute respectively (Figure 5.5), although longer grazing times (13 hours/day) have been recorded on sparsely vegetated rangeland (Smith, 1955). This gives a normal

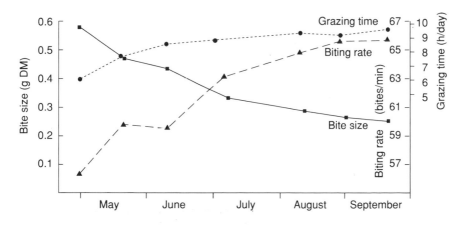

Figure 5.5   Changes in grazing behaviour over a typical five-month grazing season in the UK, during which time the herbage height declined from 10 cm at turnout to 5 cm at housing. (Phillips and Leaver, 1985)

maximum of 50,000 bites/day, although individual cattle achieve more. High-yielding cows can only achieve long grazing times at the expense of lying and ruminating times but may be reluctant to do this (see page 179). There is little else that they can sacrifice, as an ethogram for a high-yielding grazing cow demonstrates (Figure 5.6), and this emphasises the need to minimise the time that high-yielding cows are kept off the pasture for milking.

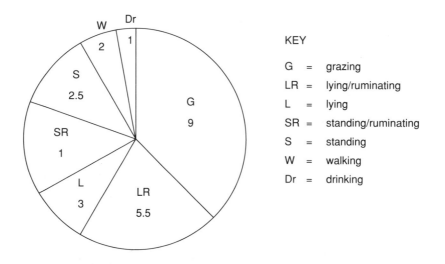

Figure 5.6   Ethogram for a high-yielding dairy cow. Values are hours/day.

Grazing lactating dairy cows typically have about five meals per day, each lasting on average 110 minutes (Figure 5.7). Cattle with lower intake requirements in relation to their weight (e.g. dry cows, mature bullocks) have fewer and shorter meals. Normally the first meal begins shortly after dawn, followed by two to three meals between morning and afternoon milking, and the longest, most intensive meal in the evening ending around dusk. This is to provide sufficient food to digest during the night period. There is often a short meal averaging 30 minutes at about 1 a.m., after which the rest of the night is spent ruminating and resting (Phillips and Denne, 1988).

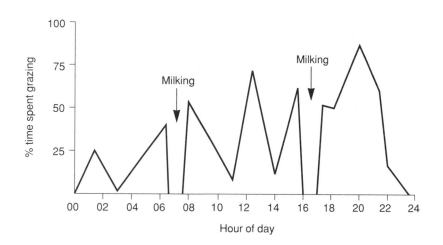

Figure 5.7   Change in grazing intensity over the day for a lactating cow.

Browsing

Browsing is the feeding on woody plant material, i.e. shrubs and trees (Plate 5.2). Many animals do not actually consume the woody

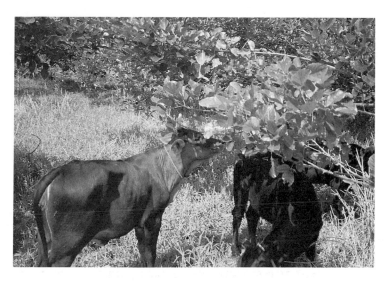

Plate 5.2   Young cattle in the tropics browsing on trees.

part of the plant but selectively eat the leaves and young shoots. Goats and many of the African ungulates have this capacity. Cattle, however, do not because their oral structure contains a broad, flattened lower incisor arcade (see Plate 7.12), whereas browsers have narrow, pointed incisor arcades with which to select leaves, fruit, etc. from woody perennials (Gordon and Illius, 1988).

Browse thus does not normally make up a significant part of the diet of cattle (Plate 5.3). However, where the browse species can be consumed without much selectivity, e.g. bamboo, cattle can eat large quantities of leaves and young shoots (Plate 5.4). Theoretically, bamboo as a monocotyledon might not be regarded as a browse species, but the behavioural mechanism of feeding is more similar to browsing than grazing. In natural forest cattle can survive on feeds such as these during a dry season, whereas goats and deer will survive primarily on more differentiated plants, mainly dicotyledons. Browse is more important in tropical countries where the shortage of fodder during dry periods is not so easily buffered by conserved feed as in temperate countries. In some tropical regions

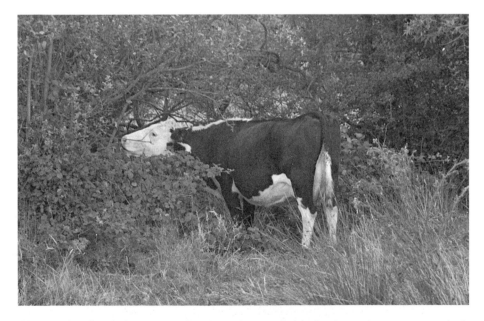

Plate 5.3   Cattle browse only when the available herbage is mature and of poor nutritional value or is in short supply.

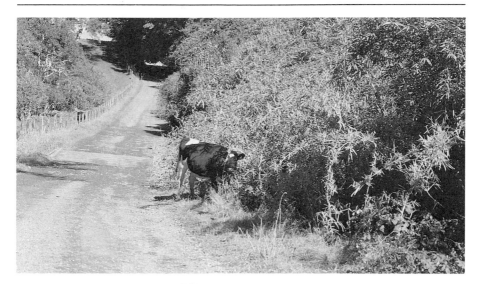

Plate 5.4   A young steer feeding on bamboo on the edge of indigenous forest in southern Chile.

tree leaves are collected manually for cattle feeding, which is the browsing equivalent of zero-grazing.

Eating Conserved Feed

Both concentrates and forages are often harvested by man and preserved for use when grazed feeds are scarce. As conserved feeds are usually presented in a readily prehendible form, suitable for large bites, the rate of intake is usually high (Table 5.2). Some conserved forages are, however, more fibrous than most grazed herbage or concentrates, and these are usually masticated for a longer period, during both eating and rumination. This helps to comminute the plant parts and expose more cells to the slow process of fibre digestion.

Many factors influence the rate of an animal's intake of conserved feeds. Lactating cattle, for example, which have high intake requirements, eat faster than dry cows, and dominant cows eat faster than subordinates. Animal size also makes a considerable difference, and it is important to remember that heifers, for example, take longer to eat concentrates in the parlour than cows.

Feed form and composition are also important. Dusty pellets or

TABLE 5.2   Typical rates of eating conserved feeds.

	g DM/minute
Oat straw	20
Hay	30
Grass silage	45
Ground and pelleted hay	80
Concentrate meal	250
Concentrate pellets	400

(From Campling and Morgan, 1981; Phillips, 1983)

meals are not eaten rapidly, and generally the drier the feed, the more saliva that is required to produce a bolus suitable for swallowing. Acid feeds such as silage are eaten quite rapidly but the meals are short, suggesting that rumen or buccal receptors inhibit meal length. Buccal receptors may control rumination by the pH of the regurgitated boli, as monitored by the tongue. Excessive saltiness or bitterness also reduces the rate of intake of concentrates, although a limited amount of salt mixed in with the feed seems to increase palatability. Indeed, it used to be a common practice to add some salt to make hay or silage more palatable.

With silages in particular some selectivity is evident during feeding. Cattle 'nose' silage and to some extent hay to find the bits that taste or smell the best. While we cannot be sure exactly what they are searching for, it is likely that feed previously contaminated or 'marked' with another cow's saliva will be rejected since newly offered feeds are usually consumed at a rapid rate. Conceivably it is pheromones in the cow's saliva which contaminate the feed, but no direct evidence is yet available on this. Often with silage feeding, 'nosing' turns into 'feed tossing' behaviour, which can result in a waste of feed (Plate 5.5). First a mouthful of silage is taken; then by dipping the head and twisting the neck upwards the silage is thrown upwards into the air, often landing on the back of the animal. Usually only a small proportion of the herd indulge in this wasteful behaviour, which is especially common if the feed is offered from a bunk or trough where the bottom is not at floor level (colour plate 16). Swallowing may be easier when the head is lowered, as it would be during grazing, but it is possible that the feed tossing behaviour is a redirected sward ripping action (which would normally be performed 30–40,000 times/day).

Whereas it is unlikely that space availability will limit the intake of grazing cattle, this is an important consideration with loose housed cattle. A large area per animal is obviously expensive to provide and can lead to abnormal behaviours such as lying on the floor instead of in cubicles. Too little space, however, increases competition between the cattle and reduces intake. Interestingly, if feeding space or feed is restricted, the dominant cows do not seem to maintain ad libitum intake by feeding at non-preferred times at the expense of the intake of subordinate cows. Either there is a strong disincentive for the dominant cows to feed at non-preferred times (a new feeding dominance order at these times effectively) or they are behaving altruistically.

Housed cattle will typically eat silage or hay in 6–12 meals per day for a total of 4–7 hours/day. However, providing only this amount of time for the cows to eat will reduce intake by about 20% (Campling and Morgan, 1981), demonstrating the need for cattle to spread their feeds out over the day. Intake will also be restricted if

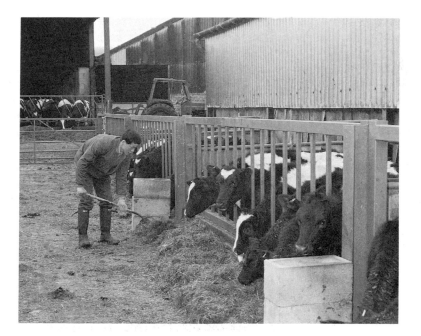

Plate 5.5   Returning silage that has been 'nosed' and tossed
is a time-consuming task.

less than 40–50 cm of feeding space is available per animal. Like grazing cattle, they prefer to take most feed during daylight hours, but there is often some feeding by subordinate cows overnight. Unlike grazing cattle, housed cattle show little social facilitation in feeding, and this may weaken the social bonds and increase tension in the herd.

Self-feed Silage

A common system of feeding silage that is popular in the UK and requires little mechanisation is for the cows to vertically 'graze' direct from a silage clamp. Feeding time is usually similar to trough or floor-fed silage, but the silage can be difficult to prehend, especially for young cattle losing their milk teeth, if it has not been chopped at harvesting to about 2 cm. In the same way that an electrified wire can limit access to new grazing in the field, an electrified bar or a solid barrier about 0.9 m from the floor is needed to ensure silage is not eaten just from the middle of the clamp. The stockman moves the bar or barrier closer to the silage face at regular intervals, thereby allowing access to fresh silage.

Care must be taken if young heifers are required to feed with older cattle in this system, particularly if access to the feed face is limited. It will take some time for them to overcome their fear of the wire, and they may also be bullied by older cows. In situations like this they inevitably resort to feeding at a less favoured time such as between 2 a.m. and 5 a.m. If the feed face is limiting, a ring feeder holding cut silage may be used to provide a greater area of access.

Eating Supplements

Most cattle are offered some form of supplement to complement the nutritional value of the basal forage or grazed feed. Often these supplements are of higher soluble carbohydrate content than the forage and tend to be preferred to it. If supplied in small quantities, intake rate is usually high; for example, silage offered as a supplement to grazed herbage will be eaten at 60–70 g DM/minute. The greater the amount of supplement offered, the slower the intake rate. The rapid intake rate of supplements is of benefit to grazing cows, which are often short of time to harvest sufficient feed. There is no ideal time to offer the supplement because some substitution for the basal forage is inevitable, however undesirable it may be economically. Attempts to restrict its availability to non-preferred feeding times, e.g. at night, have not been successful in preventing the intake of basal forage being reduced because the cow readily modifies her behaviour to cope with the new feeding times. In this respect it appears that the preference for feeding mainly during daylight may arise not so much from energetic benefits gained from adequate rest at night as be a vestigial defence mechanism to restrict grazing when predators cannot be seen. There is, however, some evidence that morning supplementation is better than afternoon (Adams, 1985). Some 'lazy' cows prefer conserved supplements such as silage to grazed grass because they can be eaten rapidly. This can even be to the detriment of their milk production; in this instance the cow is trading hunger satiation for more rest.

The rapid intake rate of conserved or zero-grazed feeds is primarily due to a large bite size (Plate 5.6). Biting rate when prehending forage is low, for hay typically 15 bites/minute, but there are a large number of manipulative and chewing bites—about 60/minute (colour plate 17)—compared with cows at pasture where these rarely exceed 15/minute.

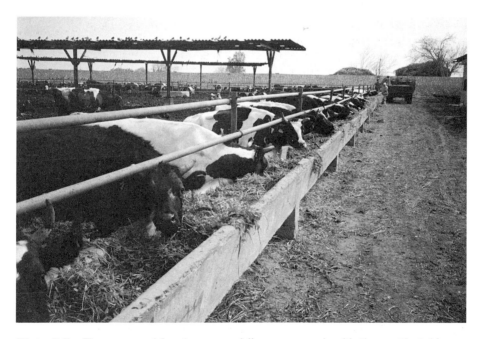

Plate 5.6   Zero-grazed feeds are rapidly consumed, with the cattle taking large bites compared to when they are grazing.

Environmental Factors Affecting Feeding Behaviour

Photoperiod and time of day

Cattle are mainly diurnal feeders, starting at dawn and ending at dusk, but when intake requirements are high or the day length is short, nocturnal feeding will take place. Cattle attempt to spread out their meals over the daylight hours by manipulating meal number and length; hence in mid summer there are a greater number of meals in the daylight but they are of shorter duration (Figure 5.8). Nocturnal feeding is more likely to occur on a well-lit night, and in hot humid conditions night grazing is increased to limit exposure to the sun during the day (Coulan, 1984). Cattle may thus be regarded as facultative diurnal feeders.

The speed of grazing or biting the pasture also varies over the day. Speed is reduced at night, probably because the cattle do not have the necessary visual cues for fast herbage selection (Phillips and Hecheimi, 1989). Some experiments have found a marked increase in biting rate as the day progresses (Phillips and Leaver, 1985). This is usually accompanied by an increase in grazing intensity, the proportion of time spent grazing. These two factors that increase the rate of herbage intake as the day progresses may be related to either the

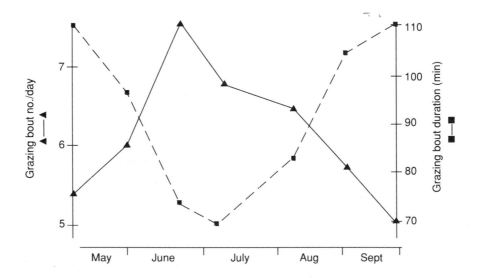

Figure 5.8   Variation in grazing bout number and duration over the summer. (Phillips and Hecheimi, 1989)

increase in sugar content of the plant over the day or the need to store up sufficient food for digestion at night.

In rotationally grazed pastures where a fresh paddock is available daily, there is an increase in grazing intensity when the fresh pasture is offered. Similarly the feeding intensity of cattle offered conserved feeds is greatest after a new feed has been provided.

Photoperiod manipulation in housed cattle can alter circadian patterns of feeding. Extending the day length will increase the number of meals but will not increase the total daily feeding time (Figure 5.9).

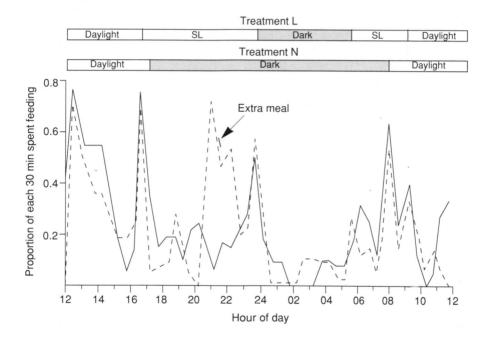

Figure 5.9   Effect of supplementary light (SL) on feeding behaviour of housed cattle: – – – = treatment L with supplementary light; ——— = treatment N with no supplementary light.

Biting rate is usually constant for most of a meal except for a reduction at the beginning and end as time spent in other activities increases (Figure 5.10). As the grazing bout progresses there is less difference between cows in biting rate. Grazing is an energetically

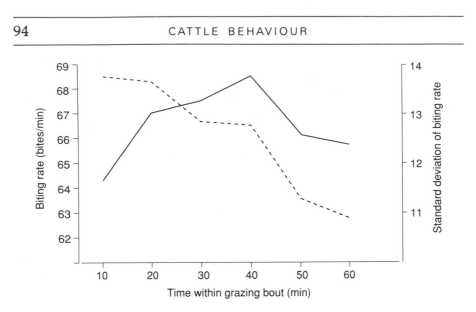

Figure 5.10   Variation in biting rate (────) and the standard deviation of the biting rate (– – – –) during a one-hour grazing bout. (Phillips, unpublished data)

expensive process usually followed by periods of just lying and then lying and ruminating. If cattle are starved for a period, they increase their rate of consumption mainly by increasing their bite size and pasture biting rate and decreasing the time spent masticating the feed.

Temperature and humidity

As inhabitants of nearly all parts of the global land mass, cattle may be considered thermolabile. However, they are prone to heat stress and unless some protection is provided their productivity falls. Both temperature and humidity increase the heat load and the necessity for cattle to seek shade during the day (thermoregulatory behaviour). Thus in hot dry conditions, particularly if there is a large circadian variation in temperature, cattle can alter their feeding times to the night and reduce the heat load. In the humid tropics there is less circadian variation in temperature, and the high humidity reduces evaporative heat loss, making heat stress a common problem. This is particularly true for *Bos taurus* cattle, which need to spend much of the day in the shade, and feed intake is substantially reduced. Often about 60% of grazing is at night, but in many countries the cattle have to be housed at night to protect against predators, two- and four-legged! This can reduce grazing time to five hours a day or less, but pasture intake rate is usually increased to compensate for at least some of the reduction in grazing time.

High temperatures/humidity that cause heat stress will also alter feed preference. Concentrate feeds are preferred, and fibrous feeds should be avoided because fibre produces a greater heat increment of digestion than other nutrients. In many tropical regions, however, only fibrous feeds are available for feeding to cattle, as concentrate feeds are required for human consumption.

The high heat of digestion of fibre enables cattle to survive remarkably low temperatures without loss of productivity, providing they have a functional rumen. Preruminant or sick cattle or those that are inadequately fed have reduced tolerance of cold stress. Feeding time for all cattle increases at low temperatures but healthy ruminant cattle can easily adjust to temperatures of $-20°C$ or below. The major nutritional adjustment that they make is to speed up the rate of reticular contractions, increasing ruminating time and the heat increment of digestion (Gonyou et al., 1979). Not suprisingly, cattle tolerant to heat stress tend to be more susceptible to cold stress. For example, Baladi cattle in Egypt, which are well adapted to the hot summer conditions, need protection in winter from the cold (colour plate 18).

Wind and rain
Wind and rain increase the feeling of cold in grazing cattle. Wind also reduces heat stress, so forced air ventilation can be used for this purpose with housed cattle.

Cattle orientate their bodies to optimise climatic effects. In cold temperatures they orientate themselves at 90° to the sun's rays (colour plate 19). In cold wind and rain they stand with their hindquarters to the wind so that their faces, which are more thermally sensitive, are protected. Depending on their degree of hunger, heavy rain may stop them grazing altogether, particularly if shelter is available, but in most conditions they will graze with the wind, travelling faster and apparently grazing less intensively. It appears that cattle are reluctant to lie on wet grass: if rain starts when they are already lying, they may not move, but if they are standing they will shelter rather than lie down. Sometimes a light shower can actually encourage lying cattle to get up and graze. The reason is unclear. Does wet grass taste better? Do they want to graze before heavy rain comes? We know virtually nothing about the ability of cattle to forecast the weather, but superhuman powers have been attributed to other animals.

A phenomenon which has puzzled farmers and scientists alike for many years is the low intake and productivity of cattle grazing lush temperate grasses during a prolonged period of wet weather. The rainfall has no effect on the rate of grass intake (in dry matter terms) but reduces the total amount of grass eaten daily, sometimes by 10–20%, and reduces grass digestibility. Addition of water to the rumen per se does not affect digestibility, so it is likely that the water in the buccal cavity reduces the efficiency of mastication and hence digestion—much as a lawnmower struggles to cut lush wet grass. The phenomenon occurs only with grass that already has a high water content. With grasses or other feeds of low water content (less than 20%), intake may be increased if water is added. Cattle therefore seem to have highest intakes of feed dry matter between about 20 and 80% water content.

Feeding Apparatus

The introduction of high-moisture bulky feeds such as silage and

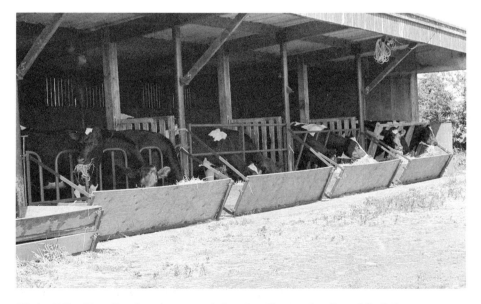

Plate 5.7   Feeding barriers on trial at the Centre for Rural Building, Scottish Agricultural College. Left to right: tombstone, rectangular, diagonal and angled diagonal barriers.
(SAC Centre for Rural Building, Aberdeen)

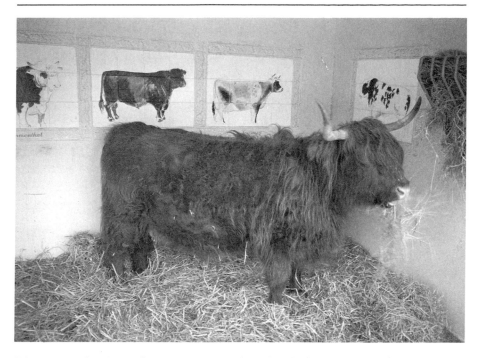

Plate 5.8   Cattle prefer to masticate their feed with the head in the
horizontal or, as shown above, in a slightly lowered position.

zero-grazed herbage has necessitated changes in the feeding apparatus for housed cattle from the conventional hayrack (colour plate 17).
The traditional feeding barrier was shaped like a row of tombstones,
designed so that each animal had to lift its head to the top of the
barrier before it could pull it back (Plate 5.7). This prevented cattle
from dragging feed out of a trough and eating it in the feeding
passage where much could be dropped and wasted. The tombstone
and other similar barriers ensured that the animal's head remained
over the feed trough whilst it ate. A diagonal feeding barrier, which
is simpler to construct, achieves the same ideal, as the animal must
twist its head sideways to move backwards. An angled feeding
barrier will more effectively contain the animal's forward thrust
from the shoulders as it feeds and provide a more comfortable
feeding position. Whereas cattle are content to prehend feed from
floor level, they prefer to masticate it with their head horizontal or
slightly lowered (Plate 5.8).

Grazing Systems

Most cattle are either grazed on the whole available area or rotated around sections of it. In intensive grassland conditions there is little evidence of major differences in behaviour and performance between the two systems. Rotationally grazed cattle, which are held on a smaller area at any one time, may have less interanimal space and increased social interaction, but this does not appear to affect production greatly (Plate 5.9). In rangeland grazing, where the areas covered by the cattle are much larger, the greater density of rotationally grazed range can reduce searching time and increase productivity (Olson and Malechek, 1988).

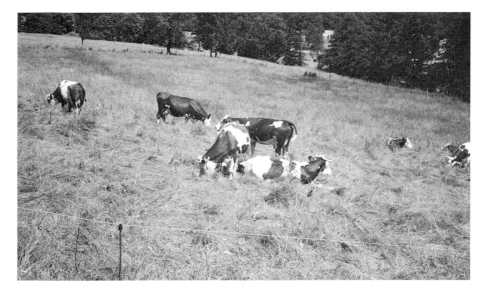

Plate 5.9   Rotational grazing can lead to reduced inter-individual distances, which encourage social interactions.

Topography
The ability of cattle to graze steep slopes is limited, and they also find it difficult to get adequate rest under such circumstances, as they cannot lie down.

Breed/environment interaction

The main cattle genotypes—*Bos indicus* and *Bos taurus*—show marked differences in heat tolerance that interact with feeding behaviour. *Bos taurus* cattle spend less time grazing and more time in the shade in hot conditions (Plate 5.10). Perhaps because of this, and the greater nutritional requirements necessary to support their higher productivity, they are less selective than *Bos indicus* cattle and have a broader dietary spectrum. Criollo cattle (*Bos taurus* cattle that were taken to South America by early Spanish emigrants) also have a greater dietary selectivity than improved British cattle (Minon *et al.*, 1984). This suggests that the period of improvement of British cattle since the Agricultural Revolution may have resulted in these cattle developing a broader dietary niche as a result of being offered a wide variety of feeds.

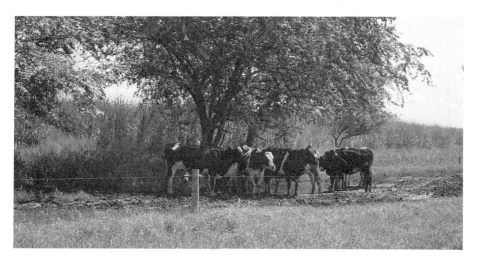

Plate 5.10   Thermoregulatory behaviour in *Bos taurus* cattle in the tropics.
Grazing is avoided during the hottest part of the day and concentrated into the night period.

External parasites

Many external parasites disturb the grazing behaviour of cattle. Biting parasites like ticks have a greater effect than flies (e.g. *Hydrotea irritans*), which merely create a nuisance. Because of parasites, cattle will change position frequently from grazing to standing, rather than lying down, and will stand with their heads facing each other. Regular tail swishing gives some protection against flies; consequently cows in susceptible areas should not have their tails trimmed. Cows also seek areas of high ground and windy places where fly concentrations will be reduced and they avoid shade, thus making themselves more exposed to heat stress (colour plate 21).

Recently insecticide-impregnated eartags have been developed which are quite successful in reducing facial concentrations of flies for several months. The normal activity of the cattle, e.g. ear flapping and grooming, causes the active ingredient, cypermethrin, to be transferred from the tag to the animal's body. Fly numbers are reduced substantially. Other parasites such as ticks may be eliminated by dipping or spraying.

RUMINATION

Rumination or 'chewing the cud' is the characteristic 'repeat consumption' process that enables cattle to digest coarse grasses. The principal function is to further comminute the plant cell walls so that cell solutes are released and the walls are exposed to microbial digestion in the rumen. An aid to this process is the mixing of the feed with saliva, which lubricates the chewing process, and adds

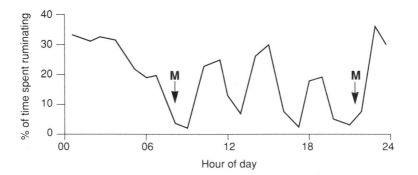

Figure 5.11   Diurnal variation in the ruminating behaviour of grazing dairy cows. M = milking time.

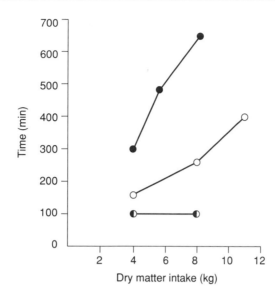

Figure 5.12   Effect of dry matter intake of hay (●), dried grass (○) and concentrates (◐) on ruminating time of cows. (Balch, 1971)

chemical buffers and predigestive enzymes to aid digestion.

Rumination accounts for a substantial part of a cow's day, altogether about six to seven hours, usually interspersed between grazing bouts and with the most intensive period being several hours after dusk (Figure 5.11). It is not a continuous process but is performed in about eight bouts of 45 minutes each per day. It is often associated with reduced alertness and its rhythmic action may induce a soporific or even hypnotic effect in the animal. It is characterised by a regular pattern of mastication, normally at about 60–70 bites per minute (more for calves). It is under voluntary control, and cattle that are disturbed and taken for milking, for example, will cease rumination. Most herdsmen recognise that only healthy and unstressed cattle will ruminate, and thus look for ruminating activity as a sign of contentment in their cattle.

The extent of rumination required for a specific diet depends largely on its fibre content but also on the dry matter and surface water content (Figure 5.12). Conserved forages that are normally harvested at a more mature stage than grazed grass are typically ruminated longer. With regard to surface water content, it appears that wet grass is not ruminated efficiently and cattle increase rumination time to compensate (see page 96 for discussion of surface water effects on herbage digestion).

Larger ruminants generally have a more efficient fibre digestion process than small ruminants because of the size of their fermentation vat (the rumen) and the ease with which stable fermentation conditions can be created in the rumen (colour plate 21). Older, larger cattle are therefore more efficient forage digesters than young cattle, which may be why they masticate slower. High-yielding cows seem prepared to forego some ruminating time to allow for other activities, such as grazing and resting.

DRINKING

Drinking is the consumption of liquids, usually water, by sucking it in through the mouth. Milk is also consumed by the neonate but this is by suckling, a specialist drinking action whereby milk is mainly squeezed out of the mother's teat rather than sucked. Water can also be lapped like a dog, particularly if there is any stray electrical current in the water, to which cattle are particularly sensitive.

Cattle need to drink at least every two to four days, depending on the temperature, the feed type and the drought resistance of the cattle. When they visit a watering place infrequently, as in rangeland grazing, they will usually spend a few hours there and drink three or four times. This sort of infrequent drinking is only found when the grazing is situated some distance (several hours' walking) from the available water.

In more intensive systems cattle drink more frequently, usually two to five times a day, although there is considerable variation between animals. Like most other animals they synchronise feeding and drinking, and for the ruminant there are probably digestive benefits in maintaining a constant rumen osmolality. Drinking is also synchronised with milking in lactating cattle, and as with feeding this is perhaps a learnt response to an impending osmotic demand. In fact voluntary water intake contains quite a large 'luxury uptake', in much the same way that other nutrients (sodium, energy rich feeds) are voluntarily consumed in greater quantities than required. This is despite the fact that some nutrients subject to 'luxury uptake', such as water and sodium, cannot be saved in any quantity in case of future deprivation, although energy can be stored as fat, which can supply metabolic water when catabolised. However, there may be subtle nutritional benefits in maintaining a high rate of feed passage, which is achieved by either a high water or sodium intake.

Most of the drinking by grazing cattle, if water is provided at pasture, is either on being returned to the pasture just after milking or during a grazing bout, often in early evening. When cattle interrupt a grazing bout for water, they may speed up the rate of walking in the direction of the trough whilst they graze or they may break off from grazing altogether and walk to the trough. Grazing may be disrupted if the cattle have to wait too long for water or if they have to make many trips for a small amount of water each time, as happens if the refilling rate is slow because of low water pressure.

Sometimes, particularly in rotational grazing systems, grazing dairy cows are not provided with water at pasture and must obtain their water supply at milking. Here a farmer must take into account the water requirements and the potential rate of water intake, which can be calculated from the weight of the cattle: intake rate (g/hour) = 0.01 × weight 0.88 (Fitsimons, 1979). Water requirements vary with diet, temperature and physiological state of the cattle. Water intake is directly correlated with dry matter content of the diet, and with very wet diets, e.g. lush spring grass, no water may be drunk at all. Normally even with wet diets some water is drunk out of habit or as 'luxury uptake' and the total water intake (free water plus feed water) varies inversely with feed dry matter content (Halley and Dougall, 1962). High protein feeds also usually require a high water intake, as do high sodium feeds: water intake (l/day) = 4.4 × 10.5 × sodium intake^3 (g/day) (Chiy and Phillips, 1992). High water availabilities are therefore very important in saline areas, where plants tend to have high sodium contents.

If water is in short supply, social factors can reduce the intake of subordinate cattle, as cattle often congregate around a water point and a dominance order develops for priority of access to the water. Intake is likely to be decreased if cows have to walk more than 250 m to water. In this case they will reduce their luxury uptake, but not their water intake required for physiological purposes.

Suckling

Both the calf's suckling drive and the cow's milk ejection reflex are innate but rapidly become habituated if not maintained. Some breeds, especially *Bos indicus*, require the sight of a calf before the milk ejection reflex is initiated. Other breeds, notably *Bos taurus* cattle, normally generalise the response from the sight of a calf to other premilking procedures such as washing and drying the udder or entry into the parlour or collecting yard. Within breeds there is variation and there is a possibility that *Bos indicus* cattle could be selected for their ability to perform the milk ejection reflex in the absence of the calf and thus facilitate machine milking. To establish a good conditioned reflex in *Bos taurus* cattle, the following should be observed: the stimulus which is to act as the signal for the conditioned reflex must precede the unconditioned stimulus; the cows must be healthy, unstressed and undisturbed; and finally the new stimulus must be benign and not upsetting to the cow in any way (Cowie, 1979).

The calf suckles partly by squeezing the milk out of the teat cistern, and partly by creating a vacuum around the teat. It squeezes the milk out by compressing the neck of the teat between its tongue and hard palate and squeezing the teat from the base to the tip with the tongue. A partial vacuum created by wrapping the tongue around the teat helps express the milk. After the milk is extracted the bottom jaw is lowered and the pressure on the teat released so that the teat cistern can fill up again. This happens about 75 times a minute for the duration of the suckling bout. Newborn calves have 5–8 suckling bouts each day. As the calf grows older this declines to 3–5 per day and the frequency with which the calf squeezes the teat declines. Cows suckling multiple calves permit a greater number of suckling bouts, up to 15–20 per day. In single-suckled cows each suckling bout lasts 10–15 minutes, but it is shorter for multiple-suckled cows. Towards the end of each suckling bout the teat-squeezing frequency decreases as the calf bunts the udder to aid passage of the milk into the teat cistern.

The calf moves rapidly from teat to teat, reaching under the udder to reach those on the far side. A calf usually suckles between the back and front legs, normally with its body alongside that of the cow (Plate 5.11). The cow often turns towards the calf to shield it. Sometimes, especially as the calf grows older, it will suckle at a right angle to the cow, or between the cow's hind legs. Younger calves often wag their tails whilst suckling, which may indicate satisfaction to the cow.

Because the calf is taller than the cow's teats, suckling is usually performed with the calf's neck lowered and the head raised (Plate 5.12). This position helps the oesophageal groove closure, where the milk bypasses the rumen to enter the abomasum directly. If calves are weaned from their mothers and given milk to drink from a bucket, the head-down position hinders the groove closure and makes the calf more likely to scour. Assistance in the form of two fingers placed in the bucket to simulate a teat may encourage the calf to drink in the head-down position (Plate 5.13).

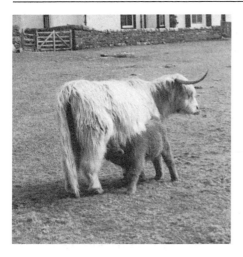

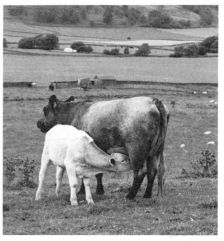

Plate 5.11 Calves usually suckle between the front and rear legs, with their body alongside that of the cow.

Plate 5.12 As the calf gets older it has to lower its head to suckle from the cow.

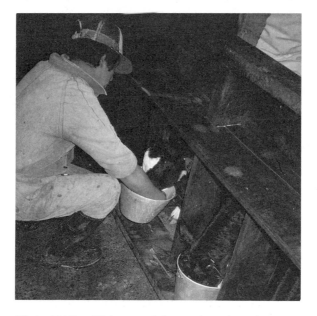

Plate 5.13 Giving assistance to calves to teach them how to drink from a bucket.

ELIMINATION

Food and water that are not retained in the animal's body after digestion are eliminated from the body in two ways. Solid material is voided from the anus (defecation) and liquid material from the penis in the male and the vagina in the female (urination).

Defecation

When cattle defecate the tail is raised and there is slight arching of the back but otherwise behaviour is not modified (Plate 5.14). Defecation may be performed while the animal is walking, standing, grazing or getting up. Cattle defecate normally about 12 times a day, with surprisingly little variation (range 10–16). The pattern of defecation over the day is mainly determined by the grazing pattern, as most faeces are deposited during grazing. Cattle are also more likely to defecate when they stand up after a period of lying, and faeces can

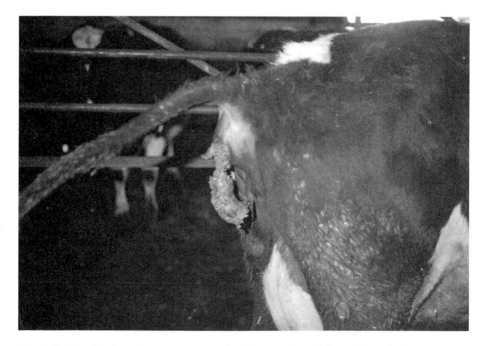

Plate 5.14   Defecation, accompanied by raising of the tail and slight arching of the back. (H. Omed)

therefore accumulate in a camping area if the cattle have one. If grazing cattle are more intensively stocked at night close to the parlour so that they can easily be brought in for milking, there may be a transfer in soil fertility due to more faeces being voided per unit area on the night pasture.

Some variation in faecal output occurs due to intake and feed type. Highly digestible feeds such as spring grass produce more liquid faeces that will cover a greater area of grass. This is often expelled further than dry faeces and contaminates the tail. Cattle that are nervous defecate more and also produce a more liquid faeces. An indication of a good stockman is that the cows do not defecate excessively in the parlour (Seabrook, 1984).

Like most animals, cattle show an element of repulsion to their own faeces, at least in their grazing behaviour. In the field each faecal deposit occupies an area approximately 0.07 m², which means that at a normal stocking rate 6% of the pasture area will have received a deposit of faeces by the end of the grazing season. In practice there is some breakdown of faecal deposits so by the end of a grazing season 2–4% of the pasture area is covered (Phillips, 1991). On average each faecal deposit causes an area of herbage six times its own area to be rejected (colour plate 22). This is initially because of smell and later because the herbage is more mature than the rest of the sward. This 'rejected' herbage will be used by cattle if there is little other feed available. Spreading slurry over a grazing pasture will also cause rejection by cattle, and if cattle *are* grazed on slurry contaminated pasture, walking time is increased because the cattle spend longer searching for uncontaminated pasture, and intake is reduced.

Several methods have been tried to overcome the reduction in herbage utilisation and intake due to faecal contamination. Conditioning cows to eat herbage near faecal deposits by feeding hay sprayed with dilute slurry or by grazing cattle on recently manured pastures has a very short-lived effect as the cattle habituate rapidly. Chain harrowing to disperse faeces and accelerate decomposition has met with little success, as it can damage the sward and does not disperse fresh deposits adequately. Covering the rejected herbage with molasses by spot spraying or a weed wipe attachment to a tractor has had some success, but the best method is to mix cattle with other grazing stock such as sheep or goats. Faecal rejection is largely species specific and is stronger in cattle than sheep, so complementary grazing of contaminated areas can readily be achieved. Zero-grazing is sometimes advocated to overcome the problem, as faeces and urine can be more evenly spread on the land at the most suitable times. The benefits for sward growth and nitrate leaching may not be that great (Hakamata, 1986) but the increase in intake can be substantial.

Indoors the constant proximity to faeces and urine in most loose housing systems may cause habituation to its offensiveness. As the ability to perceive odours is eliminated by constant exposure, this may not present as much of an offence to the welfare of cattle as often perceived by man. Deep slurry, however, will hinder cattle locomotion and it is possible that slurry which becomes caked on the skin and tail will cause irritation (colour plate 23).

Urination

Urination in the female involves raising the tail, ceasing any activities, arching the back and splaying the legs to avoid wetting the hindquarters (Plate 5.15). In the male urination can be accomplished

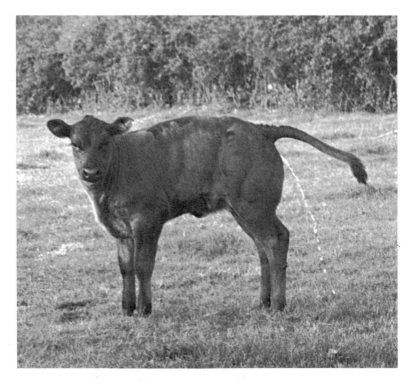

Plate 5.15   Urination in the female, accompanied by raising the tail and arching the back.

while walking. A secondary function of urination is to transmit pheromenal information.

Cattle urinate less frequently than they defecate, on average about ten times a day (Hancock, 1953). At pasture urine presents less of a problem than faeces, although herbage may be scorched at high stocking rates and during dry weather. Normally cattle prefer to graze pasture that has recently received a deposition of urine, perhaps because of the herbage's increased sodium content, and will graze it lower than uncontaminated herbage (Jaramillo, 1990).

Most urination takes place while cattle are grazing, not while they are resting. As might be expected urination is more frequent when cattle have high liquid intakes, e.g. when sodium intakes are high.

REFERENCES

Adams, D. C., 1985. 'Effect of time of supplementation on performance, forage intake and grazing behaviour of yearling beef steers grazing Russian wild ryegrass in the fall.' *Journal of Animal Science*, 61, 1037–1042.

Bailey, P. J., Bishop, A. H., and Boord, C. T. 1974. 'Grazing behaviour of steers.' *Proceedings of the Australian Society of Animal Production*, 10, 303–305.

Balch, C. C. 1971. 'Proposal to use time spent chewing as an index of the extent to which diets for ruminants possess the physical property of fibrousness characteristic of roughages.' *British Journal of Nutrition*, 26, 383–391.

Breinholt, K. A. 1979. 'Production performance of an imported herd of Friesian cattle subject to trypanosame challenge in the humid lowland tropics of Nigeria.' *East Africa Agricultural and Forestry Journal*, 44, 355.

Campling, R. C., and Morgan, C. A. 1981. 'Eating behaviour of housed cows—a review.' *Dairy Science Abstracts*, 43, 57–63.

Chiy, P. C., and Phillips, C. J. C. 1991. 'The effects of sodium chloride application to pasture, or its direct supplementation, on dairy cow production and grazing preference.' *Grass and Forage Science*, 46, 325–331.

Chiy, P. C., and Phillips, C. J. C. 1992. 'The relationships between salt, bitter and sweet tastes in cattle.' Research report to International Additives Ltd.

Chiy, P. C., Phillips, C. J. C., and Abdel-Latif, A. 1992. 'Sodium fertiliser for pasture 6. Effects on herbage composition and the grazing behaviour of dairy cows'. *Grass and Forage Science*, submitted.

Coulon, J. B. 1984. 'Feeding behaviour of crossbred Charolais cattle in a humid tropical environment.' *Revue d'Elevage et de Medicine Veterinaire des Pays Tropicaux*, 37, 185–190.

Cowie, A. T. 1979. 'Anatomy and physiology of the udder.' In *Machine Milking* (ed. Thiel, C. C., and Dodd, F. H.), pp. 156–178. NIRD/Hannah Technical Bulletin No. 1.

Fitsimons, J. J. 1979. *The Physiology of Thirst and Sodium Appetite*, p. 121. Cambridge University Press, Cambridge.

Gonyou, H. W., Christopherson, R. J., and Young, B. A., 1979. 'Effects of cold temperature and winter conditions on some aspects of behaviour of feedlot cattle.' *Applied Animal Ethology*, 5, 113–124.

Gordon, I. J., and Illius, A. W., 1988. 'Incisor arcade structure and diet selection in ruminants.' *Functional Ecology*, 2, 15–22.

Hakamata, J., 1986. 'Evaluation of the contribution of cattle excreta to pasture fertility III. Effects of aggregated distribution on herbage yield.' *Journal of Japanese Society of Grassland Science*, 32, 167–172.

Halley, R. J., and Dougall, B. M. 1962. 'The feed intake and performance of dairy cows fed on cut grass.' *Journal of Dairy Research*, 29, 241–248.

Hancock, J. 1953. 'Grazing behaviour of cattle.' *Animal Breeding Abstracts* 21, 1–13.

Illius, A. W., and Gordon, I. J. 1990. 'Diet selection and foraging behaviour in mammalian herbivores.' In *Behavioural Mechanisms of Food Selection* (ed. Hughes, R. N.), pp. 370–392. NATO, ASI Series Vol. 20.

James, N. 1992. 'Management strategies for the utilisation of high clover pastures by dairy cows.' Ph.D thesis, University College of North Wales, Bangor.

Jaramillo, V. J. 1990. 'Small-scale heterogenity in a semiarid grassland: the role of urine deposition by herbicides.' *Dissertation Abstracts International B, Sciences and Engineering* 50, 8, 3283 B.

Le Du, Y. L. P., Baker, R. D., and Newberry, R. D. 1981. 'Herbage intake and milk production by grazing dairy cows. The effect of grazing severity under continuous stocking.' *Grass and Forage Science*, 36, 307–318.

Metz, J. H. M. 1984. 'The reaction of cows to short term deprivation of lying.' *Applied Animal Behaviour Science*, 13, 301–307.

Minon, D. P., Cauhepe, M. A., Lorenzo, M. S., Colombo, I., Brizuela, M. A., and Miguel, M. C. 1984. 'Comparative analysis of diets of two breeds of cattle on pasture in the Salado basin (Buenos Aires). Botanical composition of the diet.' *Reysista Argentina de Produccio Animal*, 4, 789–801.

Olson, K. C., and Malechek, J. C. 1988. 'Heifer nutrition and growth of short duration grazed crested wheatgrass.' *Journal of Range Management*, 41, 259–263.

Phillips, C. J. C. 1991. 'Restriccion de la ingestion de pasto en la vaca lechera.' *Archivos Medicina Veterinaria*, 23, 5–20.

Phillips, C. J. C. 1983. 'Conserved forage as a buffer feed for dairy cows.' Ph.D thesis, Faculty of Science, University of Glasgow.

Phillips, C. J. C., and Leaver, J. D. 1985. 'Seasonal and diurnal variation in the grazing behaviour of dairy cows.' In *Grazing*, BGS Occasional Symposium, No. 19, pp. 98–104.

Phillips, C. J. C., and Leaver, J. D. 1986. 'The effect of forage supplementation on the behaviour of grazing dairy cows.' *Applied Animal Behaviour Science*, 16, 233–247.

Phillips, C. J. C., and Denne, S. K. P. J. 1988. 'Variation in the grazing behaviour of dairy cows measured by a Vibrarecorder and bite count monitor.' *Applied Animal Behaviour Science*, 21, 329–339.

Phillips, C. J. C., and Hecheimi K. 1989. 'The effect of forage supplementation, herbage height and season on the ingestive behaviour of dairy cows.' *Applied Animal Behaviour Science*, 24, 203–216.

Provenza, F. D., and Balph, D. F. 1990. 'Applicability of five diet-selection models to various foraging challenges ruminants encounter.' In *Behavioural Mechanisms of Food Selection* (ed. Hughes, R. N.), pp. 423–459. NATO, ASI series Vol. 20.

Seabrook, M. F. 1984. 'The psychological interaction between the stockman and his animals and its influence on performance of pigs and dairy cows.' *Veterinary Record*, 115, 84–87.

Smith, C. A. 1955. 'Studies on the Northern Rhodesia Hyporrhemia veld.' *Journal of Agricultural Science, Cambridge*, 52, 369–375.

CHAPTER 6

REPRODUCTIVE BEHAVIOUR

REPRODUCTIVE STRATEGY

Like other sexually reproducing animals, cattle are either female or male. Females produce a small number of gametes that are expensively supplied with a life-support package to nourish the fertilised gamete. Males, on the other hand, produce large numbers of gametes with only the minimum survival capacity. Given the reduced frequency of female gamete production it is logical that greater investment is provided by females to increase the chances of survival than by males. Females therefore nurture the developing embryo and provide most of the parental care, particularly in the form of lactation.

Because of their precocious development, the amount of parental care needed by cattle is relatively small, and most of this can be provided by the female. Prey animals are normally precocious to reduce the predation of juveniles. The only parental investment provided by the bull, if it can be regarded as such, is to guard the cow during oestrus and prevent her from being inseminated by a rival bull. This minimal investment strategy encourages polygyny (individual males mating with more than one female), whereas in humans, for example, the need for greater parental investment encourages monogamy (individual males mating with one female). Polygyny in turn causes competition between males for females which results in sexual selection in the males and sexual dimorphism. Sexual selection in bulls is responsible for their increased size and strength compared to cows, particularly in the shoulders, neck muscle and size of horns, all of which are necessary for effective combat to secure access to females. The dominance hierarchy so created ensures almost exclusive access to receptive females by the

113

dominant males. However, despite the intense competition between the males to secure access to females, the dominant male does not attempt to force cows to copulate. During guarding, a bull may attempt to mount and show other appetitive behaviour such as partial erection and dribbling of accessory fluid, but he will not force intromission. This is because it is in the male's interest to copulate only when the female ovum is receptive, and this information is readily imparted to the bull by the cow's behavioural signals, unlike humans where it is believed the primeval female may have attempted to hide her menstrual condition to secure greater rewards from the male in the form of food and protection (Alcock, 1989).

So far we have seen that the reproductive strategy of cattle is similar to that of most other mammals: polygynous, with competition between males producing sexual dimorphism and the females providing the parental investment. Cattle differ, however, from most mammals by being essentially bisexual, and both sexes frequently exhibit hetero- and homosexual behaviour.

Homosexual behaviour was used in feral herds as the main signal to indicate visually to distant grazing bulls that the herd contained receptive cows (Plate 6.1). It is likely that there has also been human selection for this trait for as long as the sexes were kept apart, to indicate when a cow was ready to be inseminated (naturally or artificially). However, homosexual behaviour in cows is probably more than just a signal to bulls or man. It persists even in the presence of the bull and may serve to satiate a cow's sexual motivation over and above the attention paid to her by the bull.

Facing page

Plate 6.1 Sequence of homosexual mounting in the cow.
(Courtesy of Agrafax Public Relations)

(*Top*) Initially the mounter orientates herself to the other cow, sometimes testing for the rigid back response by pressing her chin on the other cow's back.

(*Middle*) The mounter raises her brisket onto the rear end of the other cow and clasps her with her front legs just in front of the pelvic bone. As the mounting proceeds the mounter may engage in rhythmic pelvic thrusting.

(*Bottom*) As the mounter dismounts she drags her front legs over the flanks of the mounted cow, often leaving tell-tale muddy marks which indicate to the herdsman that the cow has been mounted.

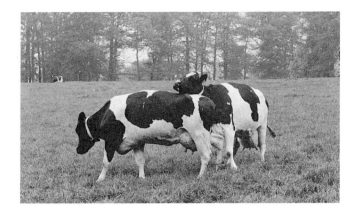

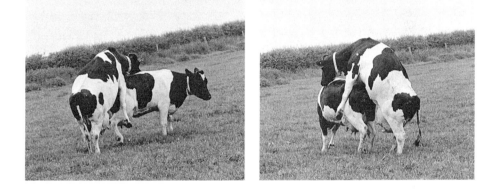

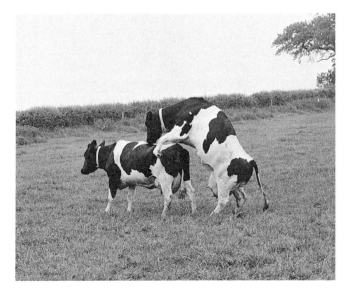

What remains a mystery is the apparent altruism in cow mounting behaviour. Why is a receptive cow mounted by a non-receptive cow and not visa versa? It may be a form of reciprocal altruism, that a non-receptive cow will expect the same attention when she becomes receptive and that the population as a whole will achieve greater reproductive potential. This might be more plausible if it were not for the fact that the mounting cow is usually close to oestrous receptivity herself. Is she not drawing attention to another cow only just before she herself is likely to need it? Herein lies the clue to the seemingly anomalous behaviour. By drawing attention to the mounted cow, a mounting cow is also drawing attention to herself and the sexually active group as a whole. Thus the mounting cow is signalling to the bull that she also expects his attention shortly, and given the bull's phenomenal serving capacity (77 ejaculations in six hours have been recorded) and the libido boost that occurs when he changes his attention to a new cow in oestrus, this should not present difficulties for the male.

In purely physical terms the stimulus for female-female mounting on the part of the mounter is an inverted U, which is provided by the rump of the mounted cow. Female-female mounting also involves pelvic thrusts in approximately 50% of cases. It is not clear what the immediate physical reward for the mounter is. Does she feel any form of satiation of libido during this potentially dangerous behaviour? The benefits for the mounted cow are more easily explained. Cows mounted by a bull experience a lowering of the electrical resistance of the skin immediately after the bull's ejaculation—suggesting an orgasm-like response (Hafez et al., 1969). Probably a similar though weaker sensation may be achieved by the rump pressure of a mounting cow, particularly during pelvic thrusts. This may be caused by pressure on the clitoris and vagina and is likely to be confined to the receptive period. Indeed genital stimulation helps to induce and synchronise oestrus via the hypothalamus. During oestrus the electrical resistance of the vaginal epithelium (Feldman et al., 1978) and mucus (Schofield et al., 1991) decreases markedly, allowing small pressure changes to stimulate large electrical responses. The importance attached to homosexual mounting is demonstrated by the fact that cows even perform it in the presence of a bull. A stimulus to him perhaps, but one is left in no doubt that cows are essentially bisexual.

Homosexual mounting in the male is most prevalent in a single sex group kept in stressful conditions, particularly from an early age. In such cases subordinate males may be excessively ridden by dominant males. This suggests that the behaviour is less related to sexuality than to aggression—a motivating force that has also been attributed to the human rapist. Homosexual behaviour in single sex male groups has also been explained, for other species including humans, as the maintenance of reproductive fitness in the absence of partners of the opposite sex. If this were the case, one would expect homosexual behaviour to occur more in the non-functional bulls in a mixed herd, which is not the case. Nor is it common in many other polygynous species, so it seems unlikely that this is the reason. Further evidence for the redirected aggression theory comes from the fact that penile intromission does not normally take place during male homosexual behaviour. It is logical that bulls should associate mounting with an attainment of dominant status, as to achieve heterosexual mounting a dominance over most other males is required. Unlike homosexual behaviour in the female, which is comparatively rare in other mammals, homosexual behaviour does occur in other mammalian males and is likely to be explained by redirected aggression rather than the maintenance of reproductive fitness.

PUBERTY AND THE ONTOGENY OF REPRODUCTIVE BEHAVIOUR

Puberty represents a series of changes in male and female animals that in cattle commence at about six months of age and culminate in the attainment of full reproductive fitness when both the physiological and behavioural aspects of reproduction function. Whilst the development of the reproductive physiology, particularly in the female, occurs quite suddenly, the behaviour development takes place over a period of up to six months in both males and females. During this period males show increased mounting activity but without penile erection or ejaculation. The purpose seems to be to learn correct orientation as the proportion of head-to-side mounts gradually declines. Masturbatory activities may commence towards the end of puberty. Mixed rearing does not facilitate reproductive behavioural development, except that the first contacts between bulls and cows reared in sexual isolation are more hesitant, with delayed first mounting and less aggression between bulls to decide sexual priority. However, after the hesitant initial encounters nature takes its course in the normal fashion. This does not imply that reproductive fitness is innate in either sex but rather that the development of the behavioural characteristics of mounting is achieved just as well in mixed as in single sex groups (Price and Wallach, 1990). The physiological development of reproductive fitness is, however, stimulated by mixed groups. In particular the presence of a bull will advance the age of first oestrus in heifers, probably through olfactory stimuli. This 'biostimulation' may be exploited commercially by using a teaser bull if a farmer wishes to have his cows served artificially.

Homosexual mounting in immature feral bulls may be seen as a mechanism to develop orientation ability that is necessary since only dominant bulls will have access to cows. In intensive housing situations, however, it can develop into redirected aggression, with the consequent exhaustion of subordinate bulls that are excessively ridden. This behaviour is sometimes discouraged by hanging electrified chains just above the bulls, but it would be more humane to reduce the intensity of the housing system or more equally match the groups of bulls. Mounting behaviour actually commences in calves as early as one week of age but develops mainly between the fourth and tenth month of age, especially between male calves (Figure 6.1) (Reinhardt, 1983). After the tenth month males are inhibited from most mounting with females by the dominant male. Males are more often mounted than females during the prepubertal period. It is possible that the tendency for male calves to be mounted by both male and female calves may reflect their tolerance of this behaviour rather than any sexual preference. Female calves often reject mounting attempts (Reinhardt, 1983), perhaps to prevent any unwanted pregnancy before they are fully developed. Male calves gradually learn to target their advances to receptive females, and by 16–18 months they have learnt to distinguish the finer points of oestrous exhibition.

Flehman develops mainly in male calves in response to females (Figure 6.1). It is common between four and ten months of age during sexual behaviour development; it then goes through a quiescent period up to 16 months, after which it increases again as males take interest in oestrous females.

OESTRUS

Definition and description

Oestrus is the behavioural manifestation of sexual receptivity in the cow. The term derives from the similarity between this behaviour and that when cattle are annoyed by the gadfly (spp. *Oestrus*).

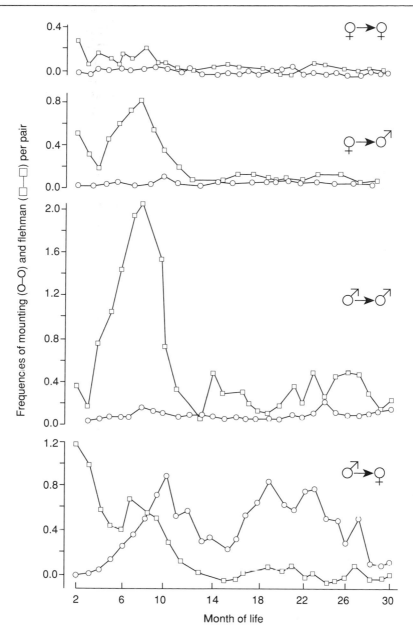

Figure 6.1 Frequencies of mounting and flehman shown by male and female non-oestrous calves during the first 30 months of life. (Reinhardt, 1983)

Oestrous behaviour is exhibited just before ovulation in cattle and is relatively short, lasting for only about 2.3% of the cycle. It is preceded by some signals that may be detected by the bull, enabling him to guard a cow until full oestrous exhibition.

A method of describing oestrous activity by scoring the cow's receptivity (adapted from Lee, 1953) can be useful for farm and research recording purposes:

Score 1   Does not attract attention of other cattle for sexual purposes
Score 2   Attracts, but does not accept attention
Score 3   Attracts and accepts attention under protest
Score 4   Attracts and accepts attention without protest or enthusiasm
Score 5   Attracts and accepts attention with enthusiasm

The oestrous cycle itself lasts on average 21 days, with 60% of cows having cycles of 18 to 25 days' duration. Cows tend to have cycles of approximately half a day longer than heifers. It seems likely that well-nourished cows tend to have shorter cycles than cows under nutritional stress (Schofield, 1988).

Oestrus is usually first observed about 50 days post-partum in weaned cows (Figure 6.2) and about six months post-partum in cows

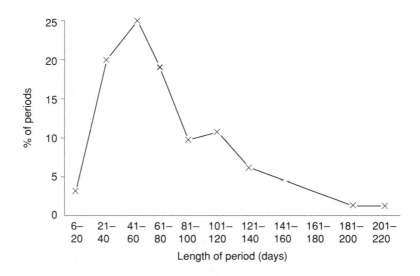

Figure 6.2   Frequency graph showing variation in the length of period from parturition to first succeeding oestrus. (Chapman and Casida, 1937)

suckling calves. There is usually at least one ovulation before this that is not associated with much oestrous behaviour. The presence of the bull will accelerate the return to first oestrus (biostimulation), as will shortening daylength.

The oestrous cycle can be divided into the following stages: proestrus, the preparatory period just before oestrus; oestrus itself; metoestrus, the refractory period; and dioestrus, when the cow's reproductive hormone output is dominated by the corpus luteum and she is said to be in the luteal stage. Of the 21 day cycle, oestrus on average only lasts for 14 hours, with pro– and metoestrus about ten hours each.

Variation in oestrous length is considerable: in one study over 33% of oestruses were less than six hours (O'Farrell, 1980), whereas another reported oestruses lasting 30 hours (Hammond, 1927). There are effects of age (heifers have shorter oestruses than cows); breed (*Bos indicus* cattle have oestruses about 65% of the length of *Bos taurus* cattle; Anderson, 1944; Mattoni *et al.*, 1988); partner (cows stand to mount longer for a bull than each other; Marion *et al.*, 1950); temperature (cows at an environmental temperature of 27°C have been recorded as having a 17% longer cycle than cows at 10°C; Pennington *et al.*, 1985); and season (oestrous lengths are reported as 15 hours in spring and 20 hours in autumn; Fraser and Broom, 1990).

Behavioural Characteristics of Oestrus

True oestrus is characterised by the cow being willing for other cattle, male or female, to mount her (colour plate 24). She indicates this by immobility when approached and a slight arching of the back. However, before mounting can be achieved the normal reluctance by cattle to breach each other's personal space must be overcome and the cow's receptivity must be tested by the potential mounter. Thus oestrus is also characterised by communicative behaviour using all of the senses.

Visual signals are provided by the standing-to-be-mounted reflex (STBM), a generally increased activity level and tail raising and switching. In addition there is swelling and reddening of the vulva and mucus can often be seen emanating from it. Additional visual signals to the herdsman can also be mucus on the end of a cubicle where an oestrous cow has been lying; dirty and steaming flanks where cows have been mounted by cattle with dirty hooves, which rub on the flanks as they dismount; and ruffling and abrasion of the rump hair over the sacral vertebrae.

Olfactory signals are in the form of pheromones released in the body fluids, especially sweat from glands in the flank and urine. During oestrus cows exhibit prolonged anovaginal sniffing and licking of the flank area. Flehman will also be exhibited to aid reception by the vomeronasal organ. The bull performs these behaviours too (Plate 6.2) but finds it easier to test for pheromones by sampling the cow's urine. Olfactory signals from the cow enable the bull to detect a cow up to two days before oestrus, during which period he may guard her from the attentions of rival suitors. To increase the spread of pheromones the frequency of urination is increased.

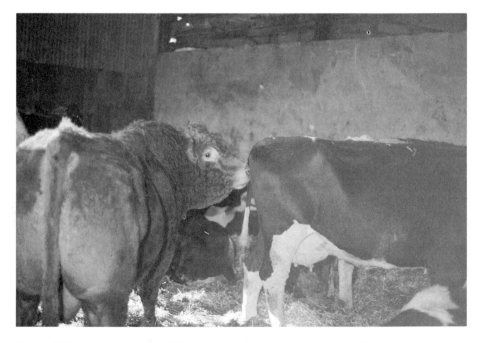

Plate 6.2   Anovaginal sniffing of an oestrous cow by a bull.

Gustatory signals are provided by the oestrous cow being licked around the vulva, which either provides direct gustatory signals or aids olfactory pheromone reception. It is often followed by flehman. Licking of the vulva may be naturally performed between cows, each head to tail.

Tactile signals are sometimes provided by an oestrous cow when she seeks out a bull and nudges and cajoles him into giving her his attention. She may sniff or lick his genitalia and mount him or other cows to attract him. She will also stand to receive chin pressing or rubbing behaviour by a cow or bull just behind the tailhead. This activity often precedes mounting and tests whether the cow has the rigid back response. Vocal signals in the form of repeated bellowing are also common.

Also associated with oestrus, but of uncertain origin, is increased aggression between sexually active cows. Although some believe that oestrous behaviour is not related to the dominance hierarchy in dairy cattle, the novel associations that cattle make during oestrus clearly lead to increased aggression. Others report that cows higher in the dominance order are more likely to mount other cows (Schofield, 1988; Reinhardt, 1983). In fact the sexual hierarchy and the space priority dominance hierarchy are not always related (see pages 54–59). The sexual hierarchy may be determined not so much by agonistic drive as sexual preferences. Like many other mammals, cattle have preferred partners, and the preferences may derive in part from such complex issues as personality and physical com-plementarity rather than superiority. Considerable selectivity is performed by the bull towards cows; he is not likely to copulate with close family members, particularly his mother (Reinhardt, 1983).

The external symptoms of aggression during oestrus may be as mild as circling behaviour during mutual vaginal sniffing and licking, but more often takes the form of tussling with the head and butting the vulnerable flank areas. It seems likely that the increased aggression arises from internal motivational forces rather than difficulties encountered in forming novel associations, and it may enable an oestrus cow to fight for the attention of her intended partner, male or female. It may also serve to dissipate the increased motivation for activity that oestrous cows possess.

Activity increases occur for virtually all oestrous cows. The average distance walked is increased by a factor of 3.4 (Phillips, 1990) but this is inversely related to the normal distance that the cow walks (Figure 6.3). If, for genetic or environmental reasons, a cow only walks a short distance each day, her proportional increase in distance walked during oestrus will be large, and vice versa. Thus cows at pasture do not proportionately increase activity as much at oestrus as cows in a cubicle shed.

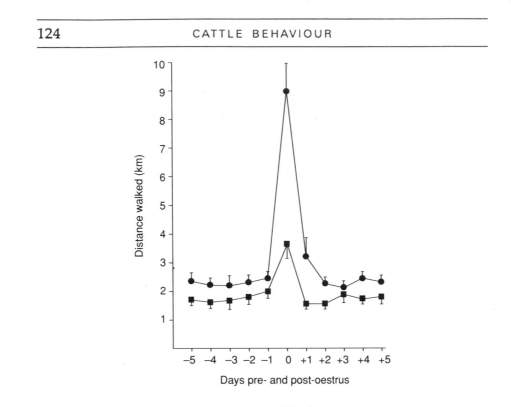

Figure 6.3   Variation in distances walked before and after oestrus.
• *= night;* ■ *= day. (Schofield et al., 1991)*

Mounting behaviour

Cow receptivity to mounting is the best indicator that she is in oestrus (Plate 6.3). However, pregnant cows will occasionally stand to be mounted by cows or immature bulls, but never by an adult bull (Reinhardt, 1983). They also indulge in other oestrous behaviour such as flehman and various investigatory behaviours.

When an oestrous cow is ridden by another cow not in oestrus, she may reciprocate by trying to mount that cow and is particularly likely to be successful if the escape routes are blocked (colour plate 25). Given these exceptions, approximately 90% of all mounted cows are in oestrus, but only about 70% of mounting cows (Hurnik *et al.*, 1975). Cows are usually mounted 50–60 times during oestrus by other cows, but one-quarter of cows are mounted less than 30 times (Esslemont, and Bryant, 1976). *Bos indicus* cows are mounted much less, typically only eight times during the entire oestrus (Mattone *et*

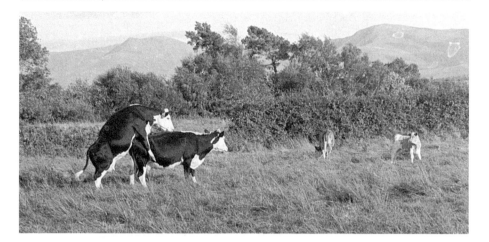

Plate 6.3   Cow mounting with pelvic thrusting (*above*) and dismounting (*below*). As she dismounts she exerts pressure with her front legs and drags her chin over the mounted cow's back, whose legs bend with the pressure. On the righthand side of each photograph a calf can be seen learning about the behaviour.

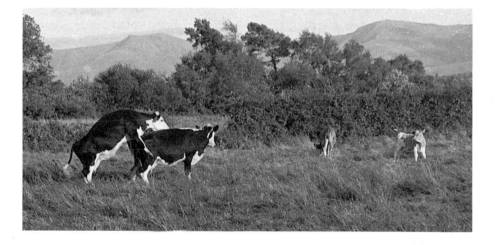

al., 1988). Mounting activity in *Bos taurus* cattle increases from a negligible incidence in dioestrus to about six mounts/hour during peak oestrus (Figure 6.4). More mounts are likely to be initiated in proestrus than metoestrus, during which time cows are usually recovering from the excessive activity during oestrus.

Although the number of cows entering oestrus appears uniform

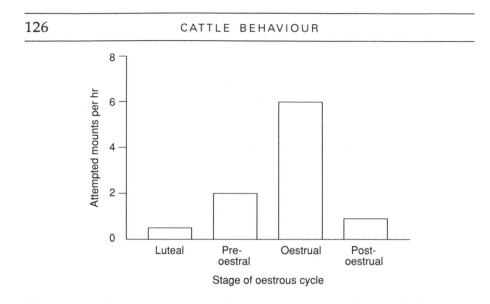

Figure 6.4 Average number of attempted mounts per hour by heifers at different stages of an oestrous cycle as defined by levels of progesterone in blood. (Helmer and Britt, 1985)

throughout the day, there is a marked peak of oestrous expression in the early evening, with some people reporting a secondary peak in the early morning (Schofield, 1988). Probably oestrus expression is accentuated at times when cows are not preoccupied with other high-priority activities such as feeding and milking but are still normally active. Management details such as times of feeding and milking and degree of competition for feed will determine the most likely times for oestrus to be expressed.

Both environmental and animal factors influence the frequency of homosexual mounting behaviour, and therefore are important in the herdsman's detection of oestrus. Mounting by the bull is less frequent than by cows and will depend on the bull's libido and the bull:cow ratio.

Environmental Influences on Oestrous Expression

Cold temperatures reduce mounting activity and alter the diurnal distribution of mounting. In hot weather cows do most mounting in the early morning and late evening when it is cooler, whereas in cold weather they do it mainly during the middle of the day when it is warmest. Heavy rain suppresses mounting behaviour (Kilgour *et al.*, 1977).

Photoperiod also affects mounting behaviour, although there have not been any comprehensive studies. Artificially extending the daylength in winter can reduce mounting behaviour and activity in general (Phillips and Schofield, 1989). As this is often accompanied by a reduction in aggression, it is assumed to be due to the improvement of the environment and resulting pacifying effect on the animals.

The physical environment that cows are kept in undoubtedly influences mounting. In a crowded building where the floor is slippery and space is limited, cows are naturally reluctant to mount each other (Vailes and Britt, 1990) (Plate 6.4). In such an environment cows reserve most mounting behaviour for late at night when the passageways are empty, which may make it difficult for the herdsman to detect oestrus. Other oestrous behaviours such as chin rubbing are not reduced on slippery floors.

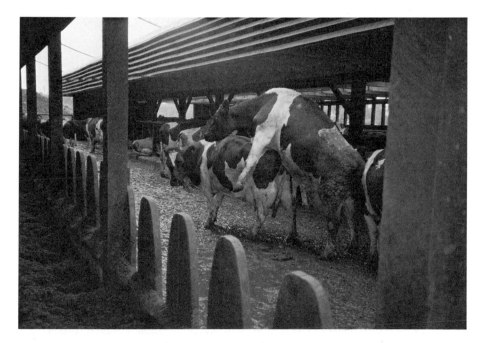

Plate 6.4   A slippery floor covered with slurry often hinders cows from mounting each other, but the dirty flanks that result from a mounting can be a useful sign to the herdsman that the cow is in or close to oestrus.

Close confinement in itself can be a stimulus to mounting activity as more cows come into contact with each other. However, mounting can be thwarted in close confinement due to difficulties in obtaining all the necessary prerequisites: other cows in or close to oestrus, a floor with good slip resistance and adequate space for mounting and dismounting with safety. Adequate space may present a problem in highly stocked yards with straw bedding. Cows usually lie down for longer here than in cubicles, presenting more of a hazard to mounting cows than in a cubicle house where lying areas are clearly defined and the passageways are free for mounting. In strawed yards teats may often be trodden on and damaged by mounting cows. More mounting behaviour usually takes place in an open yard than in a building with cubicles. Where space permits mounting cattle usually move to the periphery of the herd, so disturbance to other cows is minimised.

Routine, unstressful movement of cows often stimulates homosexual mounting behaviour. Moving to the milking parlour will often precipitate a bout of mounting, as cows are brought into contact with each other.

Animal Influences on Oestrous Expression

Genotypic differences are present in mounting behaviour (Rottensten and Touchberry, 1957) and there are probably breed differences (Boyd, 1977), but there has been little attempt to quantify these. The heritability of oestrous intensity estimated by Rottensten and Touchberry was low (0.21), as was the repeatability. It is probable that oestrus is stronger in pure dairy breeds such as the Friesian than in dual purpose and beef cows.

High-yielding dairy cows have reduced oestrous intensity (Michalkiewicsz et al., 1984). Given the extensive selection for oestrous expression in the past, it seems unlikely that major increases could be achieved by selection, and even if it could, there would possibly be undesirable genetically correlated effects, such as a general increase in activity.

Older and heavier cows tend to show a stronger oestrus than small, light heifers. The reasons for this may be the inexperience of small heifers and/or timidity at being mounted, particularly on slippery surfaces. It has been reported that maiden heifers showed 5.5 mounts/hour, first calvers 6.3 mounts/hour and older cows 7.9 mounts/hour (Gwazdauskas et al., 1983), also that oestrous behaviour is reduced in senility, which cows rarely reach (Boyd, 1977). Within this age influence, which is not strong, there are preferences for individual cows and bulls as homosexual and heterosexual partners respectively which can influence oestrus.

Nutrition does not greatly affect oestrous intensity but low-energy intakes can slightly reduce the increase in activity at oestrus (Kitwood, 1991).

The most significant animal factor affecting oestrous expression is social facilitation. A single oestrous cow in a group of cows in dioestrus shows very little oestrous behaviour other than increased activity to search for potential partners. Mounting behaviour increases in proportion to the number of cows in oestrus up to four and then may decline (Esslemont *et al.*, 1980). When several cows are in oestrus, proestrus or metoestrus, they form themselves into a sexually active group (Williamson *et al.*, 1972). Usually three to four in number, these interact together, with cows not fully in oestrus joining just for brief periods. New partners stimulate sexual activity, whereas just two cows together lose interest in each other (Alexander *et al.*, 1984). The presence of people can also stimulate mounting activity (Williamson *et al.*, 1972), provided it does not stress the cows. This may derive from the connection between imprinting and sexual preferences.

Compensatory Behaviour and Refraction

The oestrous behaviours described so far have all increased in time, demonstrating an increase in motivation. Inevitably other behaviours must decline in priority, and these are usually resting and feeding. Resting and ruminating are normally a high priority in the hard-working, high-yielding dairy cow, but during oestrus the motivation for activity, especially locomotion, is increased and rest is suspended until the metoestrous period. It is not clear to what extent cows increase their *rate* of feeding during oestrus to compensate for reduced feeding time. The potential for this is probably greater for housed cattle than for grazing cattle, where the rate of intake is determined largely by sward height. In housed cattle receiving conserved forage the number of manipulative and masticatory bites can be reduced, as well as the length of the rumination period. This will increase intake rate and hence maintain short-term satiation but reduce digestibility. In the long term, feeding behaviour will be restored to its normal dioestrous level, and nutrient supply restored. The difficulties of increasing intake rate in grazed cattle are probably greater. Bite depth could be increased by biting closer to the sward but biting rate would decline and the digestibility of ingested material would fall. Mastication and manipulative bites are few in number and so cannot be reduced, but rumination time could be reduced. The difficulty in maintaining the intake of grazing oestrous cows may be why the proportional increase in oestrous activity is less.

Metoestrus encompasses a quite sudden reduction in oestrous behaviour and a refractory period when the cow recovers from her exertions of the previous 10–20 hours. This usually takes the form of increased lying time and reduced standing, walking and feeding. These differences have only been found in a straw yard, not in the cubicle environment, because the straw yard is more conducive to long periods of rest, whereas cubicles are usually not comfortable

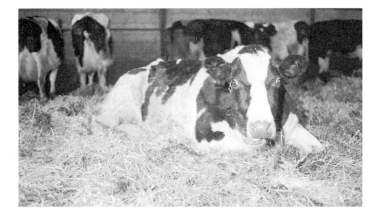

Plate 6.5   The greater comfort of cows in a straw yard (*above*) than in cubicles (*below*) encourages them to rest more after oestrus.

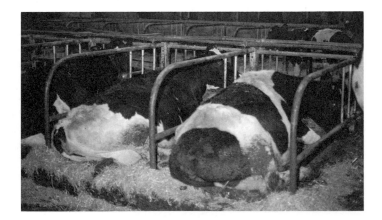

enough for this (Phillips and Schofield, 1990) (Table 6.1) (Plate 6.5).
As with oestrus the extent to which a reduction in feeding time
during metoestrus can be compensated for by an increase in feeding
rate is unclear. In any event ruminant animals are better able to
withstand a reduction in feed intake than monogastric animals because of feed reserves in the rumen.

TABLE 6.1 Time spent by cows in a straw yard and cubicles in different
behaviours on the day of oestrus (0), day before oestrus (−1), day after oestrus
(+1) and mean of other non-oestrous days (Rest).

Time spent (min per 100 min)	Straw yard (S)				Cubicles (C)			
	−1	0	+1	Rest	−1	0	+1	Rest
Lying	46	36	72	52	37	29	39	34
Standing	17	43	10	18	43	43	35	44
Feeding	37	17	18	29	18	22	24	20
Walking	0.3	3.1	0.3	0.8	1.9	5.5	1.3	1.7

(From Phillips and Schofield, 1990)

Oestrous Detection

Most dairy cows are kept in single sex groups, and the herdsman
needs to know when individual cows are in oestrus to arrange for
them to be inseminated, either naturally or artificially. Beef cows are
more often run with a bull, because of the difficulty of detecting
oestrus as this is less intensive, and the cattle are less regularly
observed. Many dairy cows are kept unrestrained in a building,
yard or at pasture and the behavioural changes associated with
homosexual oestrous interactions can be detected by the herdsman.
Observation is, however, often restricted to milking times and collection for milking (Williamson et al., 1972), which gives detection
rates of only 50–60% of oestruses. Detection rates for 2, 3, 4 and 5
observations/day of 20 minutes each have been recorded as 62, 78,
80 and 91% respectively, with the best results being achieved by
early morning and late evening observations (Esslemont et al., 1985).
As well as the proportion of oestruses missed, it is important to

consider the proportion of cows detected 'in oestrus' that were actually in dioestrus (false positives). Depending on the experience of the observer and the time spent in observation, this will be upwards of 5% (Williamson *et al.*, 1972).

Apart from the behavioural changes, the herdsman has one daily measure that may assist in detecting oestrus—the yield of milk. At the first milking after the onset of oestrus about 80% of dairy cows withhold some of their milk, and yield and fat content are reduced. In these cows there is a compensatory increase in yield at the second milking after the onset of oestrus. However, despite new parlour technology enabling milk yield to be automatically recorded and computed at each milking, the effect is not of sufficient magnitude or reliability to be used as the sole determinant of oestrus (Schofield *et al.*, 1991).

Tethered cows do not normally show any of the interactive oestrous behaviours (mounting and investigative behaviours), although they may do so if they are taken in a group for milking. They exhibit a general restlessness, vulva swelling and mucus production, and increased vocalisation. The degree of personal attention required by tethered cows for feeding, milking, etc means that oestrous detection rates are frequently as high as or higher than for loose-housed cows (Hackett and McAllister, 1984) (Plate 6.6).

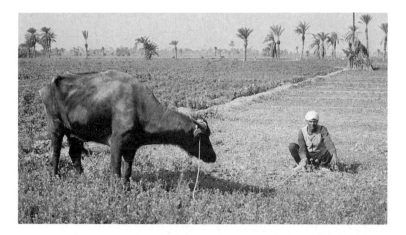

Plate 6.6   Although tethered cows do not show homosexual behaviour during oestrus, the other signs are usually readily detected during close contact with the herdsman.

Aids to Detecting Oestrous Behaviour

Apart from diligence and attempts to quantify the intensity of oestrus while recording, the herdsman may be aided in detecting oestrous behaviour by a variety of instruments.

Pedometers can be used to indicate the extent to which walking activity is increased (Plate 6.7). Given accurate information on the number of steps taken by each cow during the previous two to three days, a mathematical formula or algorithm can be used to reliably detect all cows in oestrus with no false positives (Schofield *et al.*, 1990). The high success rate of this method is due to the large and predictable increase in walking rate at oestrus and the limited variation in dioestrous walking rate (see Figure 6.4). An important feature of this and other behaviour-detecting instruments is that each cow has a characteristic rate of locomotion and a separate threshold must be established for each cow. Thus each cow must wear the pedometer for four to five half-day periods to establish a threshold. The use of pedometers is just beginning to gain acceptance, and the difficulties manufacturers have faced in designing a reliable device have been considerable.

Pedometers are basically of two types. The simplest devices record stepping rate and telemetrically send the information for each cow to

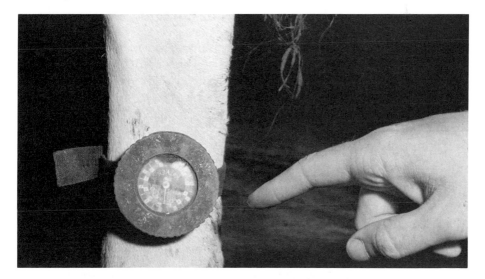

Plate 6.7   A simple pedometer to indicate oestrus.

an in-parlour recorder that is linked to an automatic identification device at each stall. In this case the pedometer can be small and unsophisticated, but considerable investment is required in parlour-recording and data-processing facilities.

The second type of pedometer is fully self-contained, and although no more sophisticated than a modern digital wristwatch, it has not yet received the same financial support to reduce its size and increase its reliability. It not only has to record step number and time, but also to process the data and indicate when the cow is in oestrus. This may be done visually by coloured lights or audibly by a repeated tone. Inevitably such a device is more expensive than a telemetric recorder for in-parlour processing, and a high degree of loss or breakage is unacceptable. It has the advantage, however, of not requiring automatic cow identification and would therefore probably appeal to the smaller farmer.

The increase in activity and other oestrous behaviour can be monitored remotely using closed-circuit television. The benefits of this are limited unless the oestrous behaviour can be automatically detected. Possibilities for this include pixel monitoring to detect activity increases or infra-red sensors just above the level of the cows' backs to detect mounting behaviour. Neither has yet been exploited commercially.

Oestrous pheromone detection is not solely intraspecific. Interspecific tests have shown that dogs and rats can accurately detect the oestrous odours of cows, albeit not quite as successfully as the bull, who can olfactorily detect the onset of proestrus. Direct chemical detection would avoid the need for expensive animal training, but oestrous odours are unfortunately a complex array of volatile compounds which cannot yet be automatically detected.

The most commonly used aids for detection of oestrous behaviour are those that are fixed to the tailhead of cows and respond to the pressure of the mounting cows. One such device incorporates a small phial of red dye inside a larger plastic container. On pressure from the mounting cow the inner phial breaks to release dye into the larger container, a change which can be detected visually by the herdsman. An alternative is a small paint strip placed on the tailhead, which becomes abraded by the rubbing of the mounting cow. Both methods are subject to a high degree of false positives as cows may rub against cubicles or other inanimate objects or be subject to mounting attempts when in dioestrus. The former device also may be subject to a high loss rate, especially in spring when the cows moult. Such methods are only useful therefore as a complement to the herdsman's observation.

Teaser cattle can also be used to detect oestrus, and they can be raddled with a pigmented marker on the brisket or chin to mark oestrous cows. Teasers are usually either castrated or vasectomised bulls or testosterone-treated females. Nymphomaniac cows (see below) can also be used but are unreliable and may exhaust themselves. False positives are a problem as cows may not be exhibiting the immobilisation response when they are mounted. Teaser bulls have the advantage that they will accelerate and synchronise the post-partum return to oestrus, but they are expensive to prepare and keep and they also present a danger on the farm. They may suffer reduced libido or develop a 'harem' of favourite cows that are served regularly (Schofield, 1988). Teasers are, however, useful if there is a problem in identifying oestrus, particularly in hot climates where it often occurs undetected at night.

Other methods of detecting oestrus automatically rely principally on the physiological changes accompanying oestrus. These include the monitoring of progesterone contents of the milk (or blood in the case of nulliparous heifers), cervical mucus conductivity and body or milk temperature changes.

Anomalous Oestrous Behaviour

Ovarian malfunction may cause oestrous behaviour to be absent (anoestrus) or excessive (nymphomania). Ovarian cysts cause both, in the approximate ratio 75:25. Anoestrus, or the absence of oestrous behaviour, is usually anovulatory in the case of cysts, or ovulatory (silent heat), when it may be due to inadequate progesterone secretion. Silent heats mainly occur during the first ovulation post-partum after which progesterone secretion by the corpus luteum allows the expression of oestrous behaviour. The true silent heat is often confused with reduced oestrous intensity. This may be caused by high milk yield, inadequate nutrition or an adverse environment, but the problem is likely to be a poor oestrous detection rate. Nymphomaniac cows generally adopt bull-like behaviour, with pawing of the ground, vocalisation at low frequency and excessive mounting. They rarely stand to be mounted themselves.

LIBIDO IN THE MALE

What Is Libido?

Unlike the female, the male does not exhibit cyclicity in reproductive fitness. In the male the degree of motivation for sexual interaction is usually referred to as libido, which together with courtship, copulatory ability and semen quality forms an important element in reproductive fitness. This is particularly true for cattle where the majority of cows are mated by just the dominant male. In this case the libido of the males may determine their motivation to achieve dominant status and the number of cows mated.

There is little evidence of a direct relationship between libido and conception rate when bulls are compared. In high libido bulls the volume of each ejaculate is reduced due to an increased mating frequency (Lang *et al.*, 1988) but conception rate is not affected (Makarechian and Berg, 1988).

Male libido can be classified according to the following categories (modified from Hafez *et al.*, 1969):

1. Avoidance of or disinterest in an oestrous cow
2. No apparent interest in an oestrous cow other than standing near her or following her
3. Licking the vulval regions of an oestrous cow, but failure to mount her
4. Attempted but unsuccessful mounting
5. Successful mounting but without ejaculation
6. Successful mounting with ejaculation

This sort of subjective assessment is usually replaced with a test based on serving capacity. Unfortunately, the procedure for testing this has not been standardised so that results are not directly comparable. Normally one or more tests are conducted that test the bull's rate of successful mounting (with ejaculation) over a certain time period, often about 10 minutes but sometimes up to 40 minutes. This test can be conducted in a pen using restrained cows that are not in oestrus or synchronised, unrestrained cows, which is more realistic but more costly to set up. The correlation between tests in a pen and tests conducted at pasture is high (Crichton and Lishman, 1989), but at pasture the bull's mating activity is influenced by environmental factors as well as his libido.

Other less common measures of libido include the number of successful mountings until the bull becomes exhausted, the time taken to first ejaculation, the interejaculation interval and the proportion of failures to mount or ejaculate. In all the tests the importance of bull stimulation is of paramount importance. Since one stimulates the other, bulls work better in pairs. Bulls about to be tested may be brought within sight or sound of the activity in the testing pen, in which case the first animal to be tested that was not stimulated by the other bull must be retested at a later date.

Male Sexual Behaviour

Male sexual behaviour starts with an exchange of signals with the cow to indicate whether both animals intend to proceed to copulation. Since the cow is in oestrus only periodically but the bull is always prepared, it is he who shows the greater seeking and testing behaviour, with the cow delivering most of the signals.

In the first instance the bull may be attracted to an oestrous cow by the latter being ridden by another cow or calling in a loud, high-pitched manner. These 'broadcast' stimuli are produced by the cow in the absence of a mate and are largely visual or auditory. Confirmation occurs as the bull receives the olfactory, gustatory and tactile stimuli at close quarters. Olfactory signals are provided in the pheromones produced by the sweat glands in the flanks and also in the cow's urine. Flehman or lipcurl is a common response by the bull on receiving these odours. The importance of this is probably largely in sexual arousal, as well as detection of oestrous cows. Soon after flehman occurs, blood serum concentration of testosterone and luteinising hormone increase, both of which are associated with the ejaculatory response in the male (Lunstra *et al.*, 1989). Flehman is exhibited primarily in response to urine sampling (Houpt *et al.*, 1989) and the secretions of the perineal skin glands (Blazquez *et al.*, 1988). It lasts for about five seconds and is performed perhaps two to three times a day by the bull. Occasionally a cow will exhibit flehman in response to a bull's urine.

A bull will also perform flehman in response to another bull, and it has been suggested that this constitutes part of an appeasement ceremony (Kilgour, 1985). The interaction between libido and social status in the bull has not been fully investigated, but it is possible that high-libido bulls are more dominant and produce more pheromones to stimulate a flehman response by a subordinate bull.

During oestrus the cow increases her urination frequency so that the bull can sample both the odours and the taste (Plate 6.8). The bull also sniffs and licks the anovaginal area frequently (Plate 6.9). Visual signals are provided by the close alignment of the bull and cow, often with the bull just behind the cow in a position where he can control her movements. This positioning also precedes mounting, and during proestrus several intention mounts (where the front legs are lifted off the ground) and half mounts may be attempted, although the cow will not stand to receive these, as she escapes by moving forwards. The bull tests for the rigid back stance by resting his chin on her back, just behind the tailhead, and rubbing it back and forth. These identification and synchronisation exchanges take

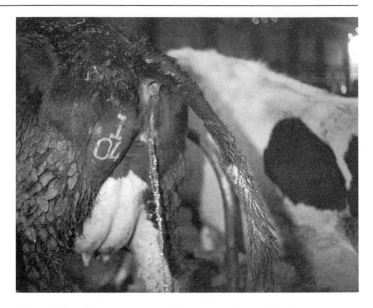

Plate 6.8   Oestrous cows increase their urination
frequency.

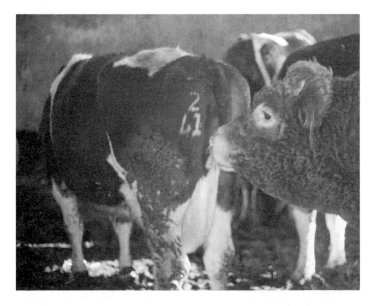

Plate 6.9   The bull is attracted to the anovaginal area
of an oestrous cow.

place during proestrus. Once a bull has identified a cow in this stage he 'guards' her for up to two days, keeping close contact and reinforcing the stimuli exchange. Direct ovulatory stimuli may be provided by the bull nosing the cow's perineum.

Finally, as the cow enters true oestrus, coition occurs. This is usually immediately preceded by vulval stimulation. Alignment follows and the bull raises his forelegs off the ground and lifts his brisket onto the cow's tailhead. Clasping the cow just in front of the pelvis the bull contracts his abdomen, bringing the protruding penis near the vaginal orifice. Once penetration has been achieved, further abdominal contraction by the bull and vulval contraction by the cow achieve maximum penetration. Ejaculation of the semen follows quickly after, accompanied by spinal rigidity in the bull and a strong abdominal contraction, the force of which may cause the bull's hind legs to leave the ground. Penile sensitivity is increased at this time, indicating that a hedonistic experience occurs.

Following ejaculation the bull quickly dismounts, drawing his chin over the cow's back as he does so. Attaching a crayon to the chin of a teaser bull (chin-ball marker) will thus mark a cow that has been mated. There follows a refractory period when the bull rests, until interest in the cow may be resumed. This refractory period varies from one to 20 minutes, depending largely on the bull himself. The coitus itself typically lasts for just two minutes, although some bulls will take longer. Most oestrous cows are served about five times by the bull, with a range of three to ten times (Chenoweth, 1983). Active breeding bulls can average 20 services per day if stimulation is sufficient.

Animal factors affecting male sexual behaviour

Genetic factors can have strong influences on male libido, which has been reported as having a heritability of 0.6 (Blockey et al., 1978). Bulls with low libido tend to have a reduced ratio of testosterone to oestradiol in the blood (Henney et al., 1990). In general, dairy bulls have a higher libido than beef bulls, a trait which may have been selected for by man. Older cattle have a higher libido than young cattle, provided that they are in good health and in particular that their feet are sound. Old bulls often develop arthritis in the joints but this does not severely affect libido or mating performance (Fischer-leitner and Stanek, 1987). Unlike many mammals, bulls are not inhibited in expressing their libido by the presence of humans or other animals. They do not prefer nocturnal mating (Crichton and Lishman, 1989), and their lack of inhibition may have been one factor favouring their domestication.

Bulls have a high serving capacity but this is usually assuaged by loss of interest in the cow. The interest can, however, be maintained by the availability of new potential partners. Promiscuity of this type would clearly be well favoured by natural selection. For the bull used for artificial insemination there is a parallel in that minor changes in the environment stimulate serving capacity. With relative ease bulls can be persuaded to mount dummy 'cows' that bear little relationship to the real thing, which is a testimony to their legendary sexual appetite. This was particularly revered by ancient civilisations, notably the Egyptians, for whom the bull was not just a domestic animal but a symbol of fertility. The high potential serving capacity of the bull is, however, perfectly explicable: most mammals with some seasonality of breeding have males with high serving capacity, and a lack of inhibitors is also favoured.

For the bull the key stimulus for mating activity is an inverted U, presented by the hind quarters of an oestrous female in a rigid stance when viewed from behind. A dummy 'cow' must be of the correct height (and strength!) and must be immobile. Older bulls are more fastidious and prefer teaser cattle, ideally female, to dummies. Sexual preparation (prolonged stimulation) is important to maximise the number of spermatozoa per ejaculate but is less effective in beef than dairy bulls. False mounts and delaying the ejaculation are methods of achieving this. Current recommendations for preparation of dairy bulls are one false mount, two minutes of restraint and two additional false mounts before ejaculation, and for beef bulls three false mounts before the first ejaculation and none before the second (Chenoweth, 1983). Beef bulls, therefore, not only have a lower libido than dairy bulls, but they also respond less to sexual preparation.

Masturbation is apparently a normal behaviour in bulls; it occurs in both mixed and single sex groups and is more common in housed than in grazing bulls. It is achieved by the bull repeatedly extending and retracting the penis through its preputial sheath and is more common when bulls are undisturbed, especially in early morning and late afternoon (Houpt and Wollney, 1989). It is stimulated by high protein diets. Only accessory gland fluids, not spermatozoa, are ejaculated, so that the concentration of spermatozoa in artificially collected ejaculates is increased. Masturbation does not confer any reproductive disadvantage on the bull and may serve to maintain reproductive fitness during periods when the male libido is not satiated by receptive females.

PARTURIENT BEHAVIOUR

Parturition is a critical stage in the bovine reproductive cycle (Plate 6.10). It involves separation of the calf from its intimate connection to the cow, and an increased risk of cow and calf mortality. In the domestic animal the risks occur in prepartum damage to the foetus, expulsion of the calf through the pelvic girdle, failure of the calf to maintain its immune status through the postpartum ingestion of colostrum, and postpartum stealing of the calf by another cow. In feral cattle there was the added danger of predation of the neonate, which is particularly vulnerable until it is reasonably mobile.

Early signs of impending parturition may sometimes be detected six weeks prepartum, when cows avoid aggressive interaction with other cattle, presumably to protect the foetus. This continues for a month or so and the cow is increasingly reluctant to engage in social encounters. She may even feed by herself or at the edge of a grazing herd. Then one to two weeks before parturition there is an increase in restlessness which intensifies in the last day or two. This restlessness includes looking and turning around, calling, licking and pawing the bedding material, tail waving, frequent alternation of lying and standing and interrupted eating patterns (Metz and Metz, 1987). At the same time there are morphological changes such as swelling of the udder and vulva and relaxation of the pelvic ligaments.

Finally the cow enters *Stage one* of the parturition itself, which is characterised by cervical dilation and ends in the breaking of the waterbag and (in a normal presentation) the appearance of the calf's hooves. During this first stage tail raising and waving is common and usually occurs for at least two minutes each time (Schilling and Hartwig, 1984). The first stage normally lasts just over two hours (Table 6.2), but in heifers requiring help during calf expulsion it is considerably longer. This is probably because heifers are more likely to experience difficulties in expelling the calf through the pelvic girdle, whereas cows are more likely to require help for other reasons, such as malpresentation or premature exhaustion.

Stage two of parturition—expulsion of the calf—normally takes about one hour. Initially the cow may be standing but she normally lies down to expel the head and shoulders. Usually she is laterally recumbent (on her side) and the two top legs are in the air. If the cow is frequently disturbed she often stands, and this can delay the labour. Uterine contractions during the second stage occur at regular intervals, usually every 15–20 minutes. Coinciding with these is a

Plate 6.10   Parturition in a buffalo cow. (M. Yousef)

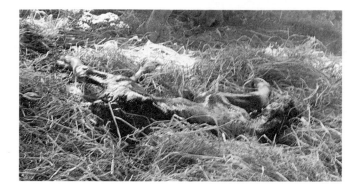

The expelled calf normally remains recumbent for
15–30 minutes.

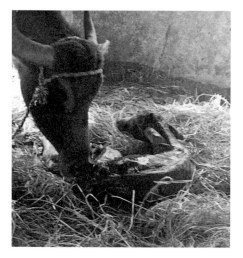

Vigorous nosing and licking by the
cow encourages activity by the calf.

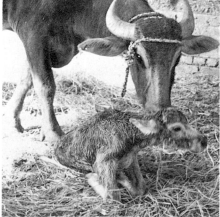

First attempts at standing are also
aided by the cow.

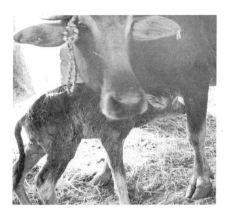

Teat-seeking behaviour. The calf is attracted to the junction of the legs and the body. This time the calf directs its search to the wrong end.

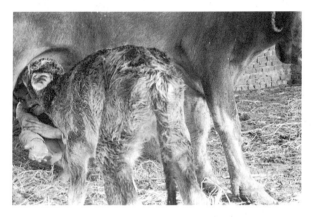

The herdsman offers assistance by directing the calf's head to the teats.

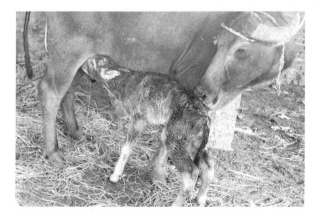

Further assistance is given by expressing milk from the teat. The cow sniffs the rear end of the calf.

TABLE 6.2 Duration of stages of parturition of cows and heifers, with and without help. Obstetric help was provided from 70 minutes after rupture of the amnion.

	Stage One (preparatory stage)	Stage Two (calf expulsion)	Stage Three (placental expulsion)
		(minutes)	
Cows			
Without help	146	64	270
With help	142	81	380
Heifers			
Without help	131	61	} 324
With help	231	96	

(After Schilling and Hartwig, 1984)

strong abdominal straining to contract the diaphragm behind the calf and force it through the birth canal. The expulsion of the head is a critical point, and once this is accomplished the trunk follows quite quickly. Difficulties in expelling the calf are one of the main obstacles to genetic improvement of beef production, since the most efficient system is one where a large sire is mated to a small dam but this often causes dystocia. Attempts to overcome this with routine Caesarean section have met with resistance on the grounds that the cow's welfare is compromised.

The timing of the second stage is important because herdsmen prefer cows to calve during the day so that they can keep an eye on them. In fact the timing of parturition probably occurs naturally at random throughout the 24 hours of the day. However, there is some evidence that cows can control it to avoid milking times (Edwards, 1979). Late evening feeding is reported to increase the number of night births (Yarney *et al.*, 1979), probably because the disturbance to the cows causes an increased risk of the waterbag breaking or uterine contractions intensifying. At the end of stage two when the calf has been expelled, the cow usually stands up and licks her calf. Vocalisation between cow and calf helps to cement the bond that is formed. Grooming may last for one and a half hours and it is in the first three hours after birth that the calf is imprinted onto the cow. Normally the calf remains passive for the first half hour, but then attempts to stand, often aided by the vigorous nosing of the cow.

If the delivery has been difficult the calf may be anoxic and lethargic and may also suffer from neonatal acidosis. The cow attempts to overcome this by increased licking of the calf (Metz and Metz, 1987). If the cow herself is exhausted this will often by done in the lying position.

Once the calf has stood, it automatically starts to search for an inverted right angle. This it usually finds in the union of the cow's trunk and her leg, and this directs it to the udder. It is not necessarily the hind leg that the calf finds, but the cow positions her body alongside that of the calf and pointing in the opposite direction so that the calf is directed to the rear end. If the cow has a large, pendulous udder the time taken to find the teat and obtain milk is about twice as long as the usual 20 minutes.

If the delivery has been difficult, the time taken by the calf to attempt to stand, to actually stand and to find the teat is considerably lengthened (Table 6.3). Assistance by the herdsman has little detrimental effect.

Some cows are not good mothers and may either show aggression to the calf or pay it little attention. There is some evidence that the rearing environment of the cow may influence her maternal instinct (Donaldson, 1970).

The final stage (*Stage three*) of parturition is the passing of the

TABLE 6.3 Duration of time intervals between birth and the start of various activities in calves whose mothers received varying degrees of assistance during delivery.

	Without help	With help from herdsman	Difficult delivery*
		(minutes postpartum)	
First attempt to stand up	13	16	29
First stood up	45	50	164
First looking for udder	65	62	> 240
First suckling	116	131	> 240

* Supervision by a veterinarian required either because hooves did not appear at the end of Stage One or traction by the herdsman was not sufficient to allow the cow to expel the calf.

(After Metz and Metz, 1987)

placenta, generally four to six hours postpartum. The cow usually eats this, and often the bedding contaminated with foetal and placental fluids. Calves in the wild are usually hidden, rather than following their dam as lambs do. In 'hider' species the dam eats the placenta to remove any traces of the birth that might attract predators, whereas in 'follower' species she usually does not.

REFERENCES

Alcock, J. 1989. *Animal Behaviour. An Evolutionary Approach.* Sinauer Associates, Massachusetts.

Alexander, T. J., Senger, P. L., Rosenberger, J. L., and Hagen, D. R. 1984. 'The influence of the stage of the oestrous cycle and novel cows upon mounting activity of dairy cattle.' *Journal of Animal Science*, 59, 1430–1439.

Anderson, J. 1944. 'The periodicity and duration of oestrus in Zebu and Grade cattle.' *Journal of Agricultural Science*, 34, 57–68.

Arnold, G. W. 1985. 'Nursing and maternal care.' Ch 28 in *Ethology of Farm Animals* (ed. Fraser, A. F.), pp. 349–346.

Blazquez, N. B., French, J. M., Long, S. E., and Perry, G. C. 1988. 'A pheromonal function for the perineal skin glands in the cows.' *Veterinary Record*, 123, 49–50.

Blockey, M. A. de B, Straw, W. M., and Jones, L. P. 1978. 'Heritability of serving capacity and scrotal circumference in beef bulls.' Abstract No. 92, 70th Annual Meeting American Society of Animal Science, East Lansing, Michigan.

Boyd, H. 1977. 'Anoestrus in cattle.' *Veterinary Record*, 100, 150–153.

Chapman, A. M., and Casida, L. E. 1937. 'Analysis of variation in the sexual cycle and some of its component phases with special reference to cattle.' *Journal of Agricultural Research*, 54, 417.

Chenoweth, P. J. 1983. 'Sexual behaviour of the bull: a review.' *Journal of Dairy Science*, 66, 173–179.

Cowie, A.T. 1979. 'Anatomy and physiology of the udder.' Ch. 6 in *Machine Milking* (ed. Thiel, C. C., and Dodd, F. H.), pp. 156–178. NIRD, Hannah Technical Bulletin No. 1.

Crichton, J. S., and Lishman, A.W. 1989. 'Factors influencing sexual behaviour of young Bos indicus bulls under pen and pasture mating conditions.' *Applied Animal Behaviour Science*, 21, 281–292.

Donaldson, S. L. 1970. 'The effects of early feeding and rearing experience on social maternal and milking parlour behaviour in dairy cattle.' PhD thesis, Purdue University, Indiana.

Edwards, S. A. 1979. 'The timing of parturition in dairy cattle.' *Journal of Agricultural Science, Cambridge*, 93, 359–363.

Esslemont, R. J., and Bryant, M. J. 1976. 'Oestrous behaviour in a herd of dairy cows.' *Veterinary Record*, 99, 472–475.

Esslemont, R. J., Glencross, R. G., Bryant, M. J., and Pope, G. S. 1980. 'A quantitative study of pre-ovulatory behaviour in cattle.' *Applied Animal Ethology*, 6, 1–17.

Feldman, R., Aizinbud, E., Schindler, H., and Broda, H. 1978. 'The electrical conductivity inside the bovine vaginal wall.' *Animal Production*, 26, 61–65.

Fischerleitner, F., and Stanek, C. 1987. 'Arthritic lesions in the digital, carpal and tarsal joints of AI bulls and their influence on sexual behaviour and semen production.' *Wiener Tierarztliche Monatsschrift*, 74, 157–163.

Fraser, A. F., and Broom, D.M. 1990. *Farm Animal Behaviour and Welfare*. 3rd ed. 437 pp. Baillière Tindall, London.

Gwazdauskas, F. C., Lineweaver, J. A., and McGilliard, M. L. 1983. 'Environmental and management factors affecting oestrous activity in dairy cattle.' *Journal of Dairy Science*, 66, 1510–1514.

Hackett, A. J., and McAllister, A. J. 1984. 'Onset of oestrus in dairy cows maintained indoors year-round.' *Journal of Dairy Science*, 67, 1793–1797.

Hafez, E. S. E., Schwein, M. W., and Ewbank, R. 1969. 'The behaviour of cattle.' In *The Behaviour of Domestic Animals* (ed. Hafez, E. S. E.), pp. 235–295. Baillière Tindall and Cassell, London.

Hammond, J. A., 1927. *The Physiology of Reproduction in the Cow*. Cambridge University Press, London.

Henney, S. R., Killian, G. J., and Denver, D. R. 1990. 'Libido, hormone concentrations in blood plasma and semen characteristics in Holstein bulls.' *Journal of Animal Science*, 68, 2784–2792.

Houpt, K. A., and Wollney, G. 1989. 'Frequency of masturbation and time budgets of dairy bulls used for semen production.' *Applied Animal Behaviour Science*, 24, 217–225.

Houpt, K. A., Rivera, W., and Glickstein, L. 1989. 'The flehman response of bulls and cows.' *Theriogenology*, 32, 343–350.

Hurnik, J. F., King, G. J., and Robertson, H. A. 1975. 'Oestrus and related behaviour in post partum Holstein cows.' *Applied Animal Ethology*, 2, 55.

Kilgour, R. 1985. 'Libido—the sexual responsiveness of male farm animals.' In *Ethology of Farm Animals* (ed. Fraser, A. F.), pp. 313–322.

Kitwood, S. E. 1991. 'Studies of the relationship between nutrition and fertility in the dairy cow.' PhD thesis, University College of North Wales, Bangor.

Lang, H., Preisinger, R., and Kalm E. 1988. (Analysis of data on semen quality in Angeln cattle obtained from a breeding programme.) *Zuchthygiene*, 23, 10–18.

Lee, D. H. K. 1953. *Manual of field studies on the heat tolerance of domestic animals*. Food and Agriculture Organisation Paper No. 38. FAO, Rome.

Lunstra, D. D., Boyd, G. W., and Corah, L. R., 1989. 'The effects of natural mating stimuli on serum luteinising hormones testosterone and oestradiol—17 beta in yearling beef bulls.' *Journal of Animal Science*, 67, 3277–3288.

Macharechian, M., and Berg, R. T 1988. *Natural service fertility of bulls in pasture*. Agriculture and Forestry Bulletin, University of Alberta, Special Issue, pp. 10–12.

Marian, G. B., Smith, V. R., Wiley, J. E., and Barrett, G. R. 1950. 'The effect of sterile copulation on time of ovulation in dairy heifers.' *Journal of Dairy Science*, 33, 885–889.

Mattoni, M., Mukasa-Mugerwa, E., Cecchini, G., and Sovani S. 1988. 'The reproductive performance of East African (Bos indicus) zebu cattle in Ethiopia. I. Estrous cycle length, duration, behaviour and ovulation time.' *Theriogenology*, 30, 961–971.

Metz, J., and Metz, J. H. M. 1987. 'Behavioural phenomena related to normal and difficult deliveries in dairy cows.' *Netherlands Journal of Agricultural Science*, 35, 87–101.

Michalkiewicsz, M., Brzozowski, P., Korwin-Kossakowski, J. 1984. 'Estrus manifestation in relation to milk yield, post-partum period, age and milk progesterone levels in dairy cows.' In *Proceedings of the 10th International Congress on Animal Reproduction and Artificial Insemination*, Illinois, USA.

O'Farrell, R. J. 1978. 'Heat detection—an observation problem.' *Food and Farm Research*, 9, 95–97.

Pennington, J. A., Albright, J. L., Diekman, M. A., and Callahan, C. 1985. 'Sexual activity of Holstein cows: seasonal effects.' *Journal of Dairy Science*, 68, 3023–3030.

Phillips, C. J. C., and Schofield, S. A. 1989. 'The effect of supplementary light on the production and behaviour of dairy cows.' *Animal Production*, 48, 293–303.

Phillips, C. J. C. 1990. 'Pedometric analysis of cattle locomotion.' In *Update in Cattle Lameness* (ed. Murray, R. D.), Proceedings of the VIth International Symposium on Diseases of the Ruminant Digit, pp. 163–176. British Cattle Veterinary Association, Liverpool.

Price, E. O., and Wallach, S. J. R. 1990. 'Rearing bulls with females fails to enhance sexual performance.' *Applied Animal Behaviour Science*, 26, 339–347.

Reinhardt, V. 1983. 'Flehman, mounting and copulation among members of a semi-wild cattle herd.' *Animal Behaviour*, 31, 641–650.

Rottensten, K., and Tovehberry, R. W. 1957. 'Observations on the degree of expression of oestrus in cattle.' *Journal of Dairy Science*, 40, 1457–1465.

Schilling, E., and Hartwig, H. H. 1984. 'Behaviour in cows before and during parturition.' In *Proceedings of International Conference on Applied Ethology in Farm Animals* (ed. Unshelm, J., Van Putten, G., and Zeeb, K.), pp. 391–394. Kiel, Germany.

Schofield, S. A., 1988. *Oestrus in dairy cows*. Technical Report No. 3. Dairy Research Unit, University of Wales, Bangor.

Schofield, S. A., Phillips, C. J. C., and Owens, A. R. 1991. 'Variation in the milk production, activity rate and electrical impedance of cervical mucus over the oestrous period of dairy cows.' *Animal Reproduction Science*, 24, 231–248.

Vailes, L. D., and Britt, J. H. 1990. 'The influence of footing surface on mounting and other sexual behaviours of oestral Holstein cows.' *Journal of Animal Science*, 68, 2333–2338.

Williamson, N. B., Morris, R. S., Blood, D. C. *et al.* 1972. 'A study of oestrus detection methods in a large commercial herd.' *Veterinary Record* 91, 50–62.

Yarney, T. A., Rahnefield, G. W., and Konefal, G. 1979. 'Time of day of parturition in beef cows.' *Canadian Journal of Animal Science*, 59, 836.

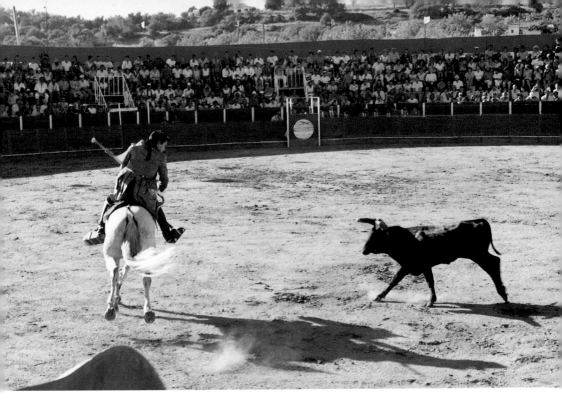

1 A confident approach by a young bull, with legs thrusting forward and head retracted. Contrast with Plate 2.1, page 23.

2 Licking by the mother reinforces the maternal bond.

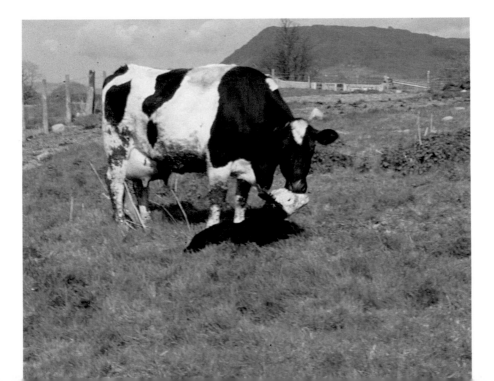

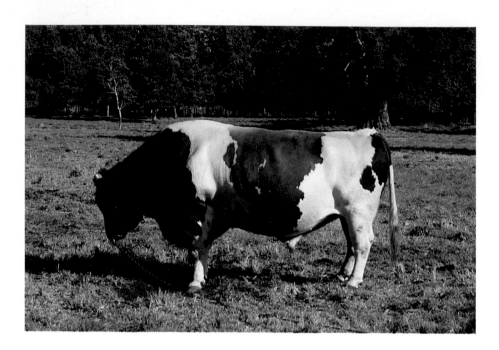

3 Threat posture in a bull.

4 Homosexual mounting can indicate sexual receptivity to cattle grazing some distance away.

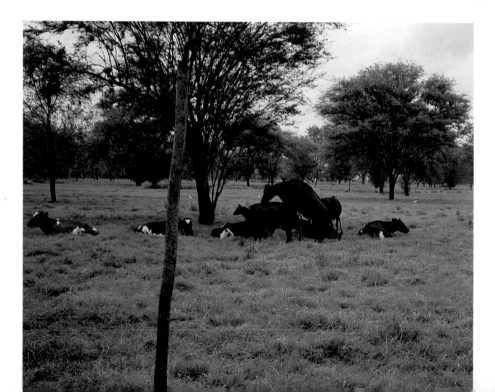

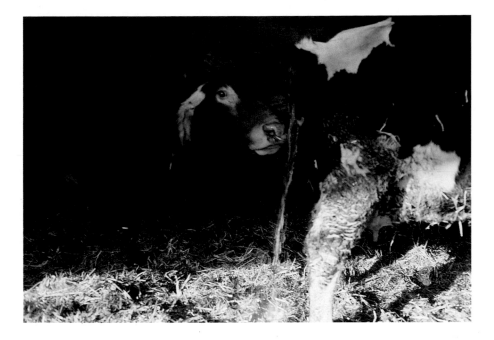

5   Bulls sniff and may even sample a cow's urine to detect hormones.

6   Cows locked in head to head combat, with splayed hind legs to increase their stability. (I. Rind)

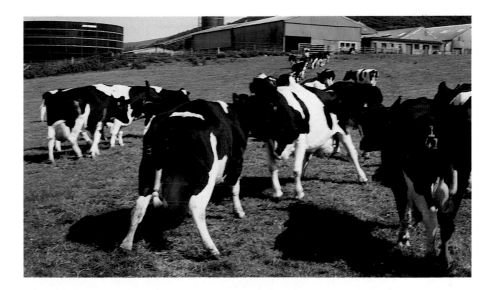

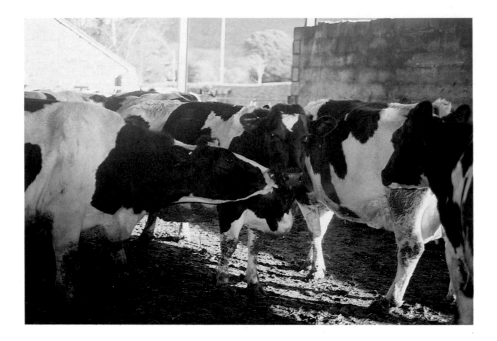

7   Allogrooming in intensively housed dairy cows. The licking cow is often slightly subordinate to the licked cows, and the body posture resembles a submissive display, thereby functioning to confirm dominance status between these two cows.

8   In many developing countries the stockman is working closely with the cattle in his care, which creates a stronger bond, whereas in intensive · production systems the herdsman is more distant to the cattle.

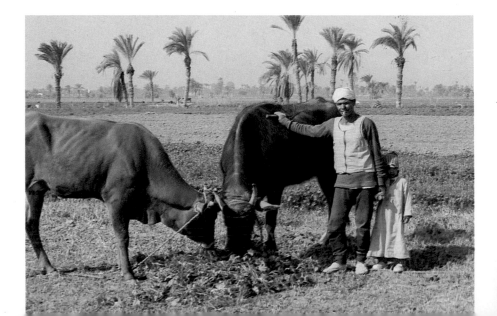

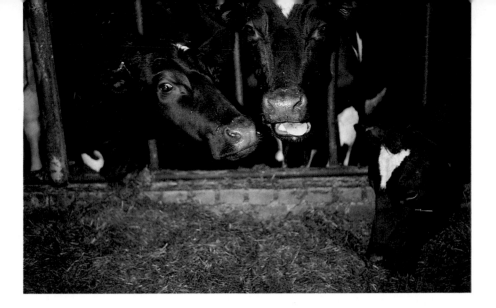

9   The close proximity of cattle feeding at a barrier encourages competitive
    interaction.

10   In most cattle production systems today the bull is either replaced
     altogether by artificial insemination or is kept singly with a harem of
     cows.

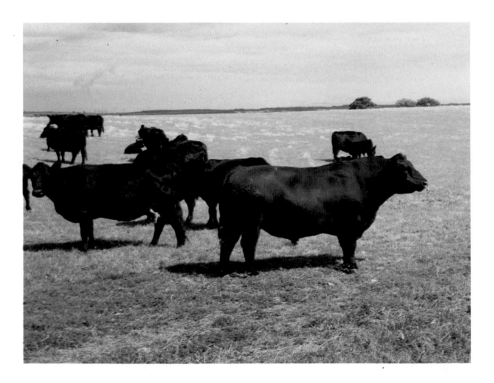

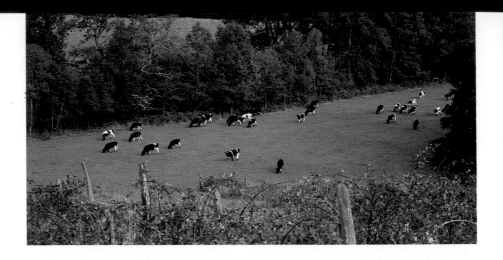

11 Cattle keep a uniform distance from each other when grazing (*above*). When they reach the end of a field (*below*) the leaders graze round in a fairly tight circle.

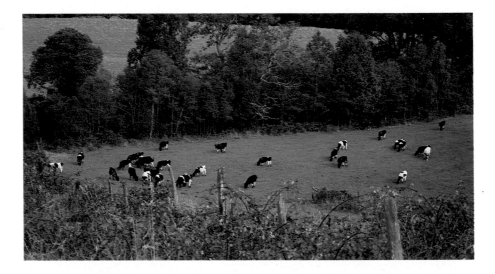

12 The flight distance is the distance that someone can approach before the animal starts to move away. In dairy cows it is usually about 2 metres.

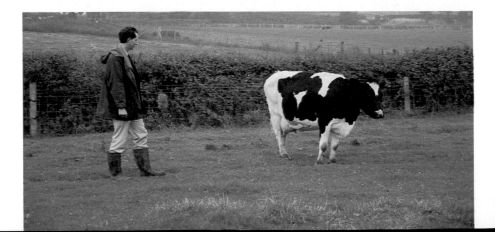

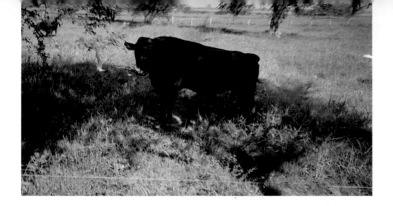

13 Shade seeking behaviour may be solitary (*above*) or small group (*below*) behaviour.

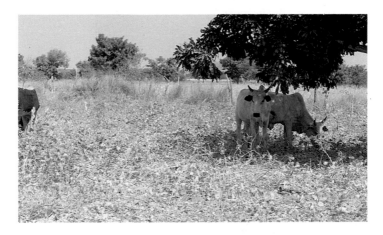

14 Cattle grazing maize stover in the tropics. (J. Shehu)

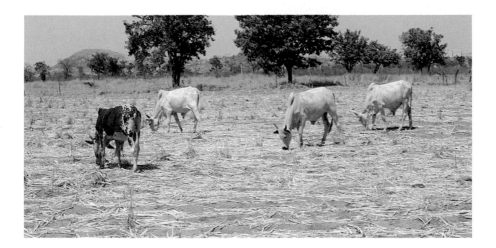

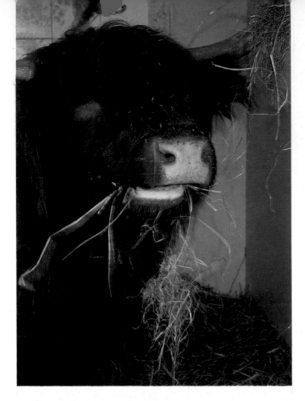

15 Feed is masticated by grinding between the upper and lower molars on either side of the jaw.

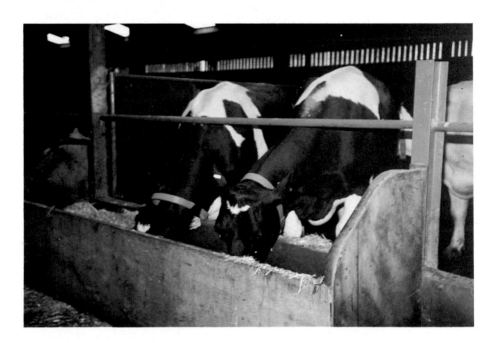

16 Feeding forage in a low trough prevents it being thrown out over the floor, and a neck rail prevents it being tossed over the cows' backs.

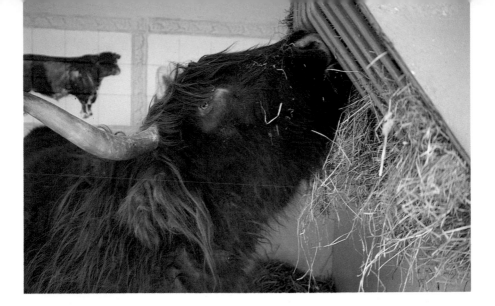

17 Cattle eating hay spend little time actually prehending or removing it from the rack or trough, but considerable time manipulating it in the mouth and chewing it.

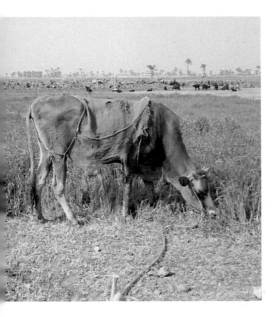

18 Cattle that have evolved heat tolerance are more susceptible to cold stress. Baladi cattle in Egypt are provided with a hessian cover during winter, when minimum temperatures are about 5°C.

19 In cold conditions, outdoor cattle orientate their bodies at 90° to the sun's rays.

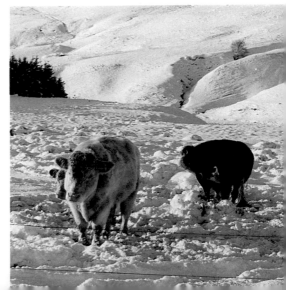

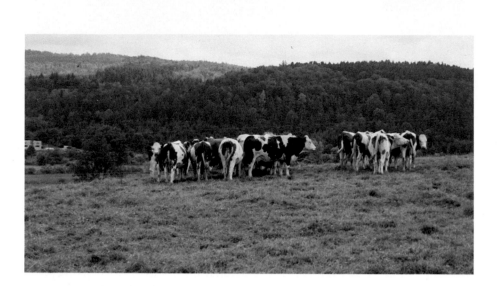

20 Cattle bunching in an exposed place to avoid the attention of the nuisance fly, *Hydrotea irritans*.

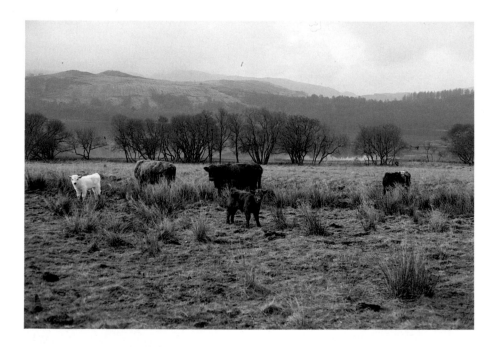

21 Cattle evolved as efficient digesters of coarse, fibrous grasses.

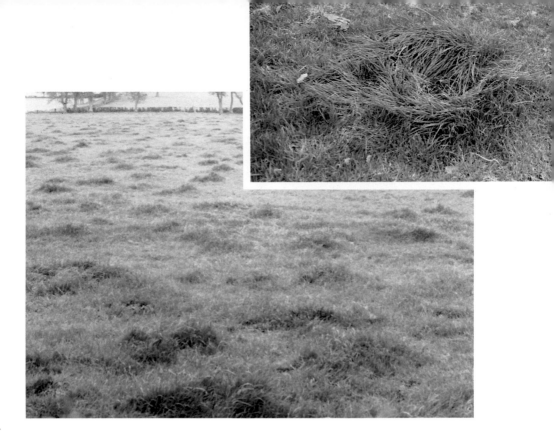

22 Rejection of the grass around faeces by cattle creates a mosaic of
   long and short grass by the end of the grazing season.

23 Keeping cattle in deep mud and slurry hinders locomotion and reduces
   their welfare.

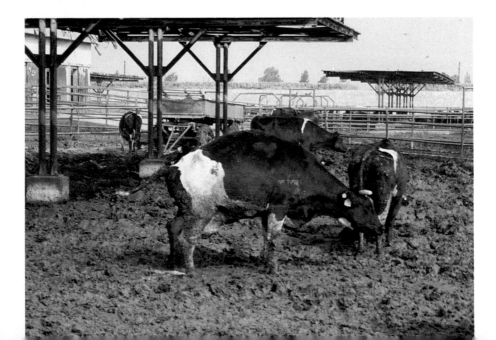

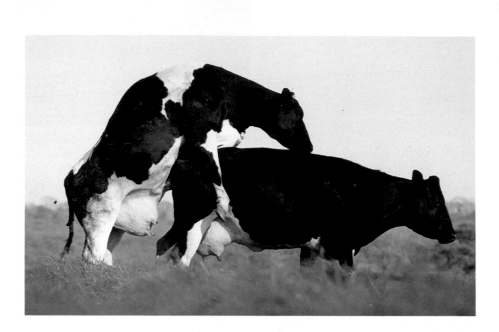

24   During oestrus the receptive cow allows herself to be mounted by another cow. (Genus/David Platt)

25   Unsuccessful mounting behaviour, as demonstrated by the escape attempt of the mounted cow. (Nicholas Spurling)

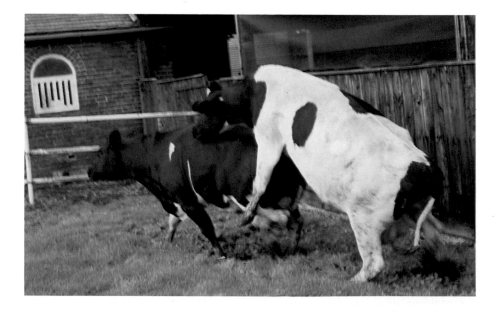

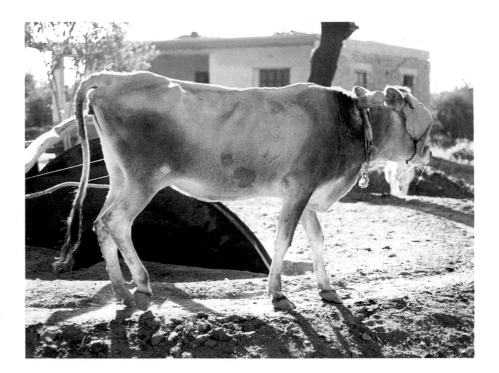

26 The walk in a draught heifer. Walking is an asymmetrical gait where the front and hind feet act independently.

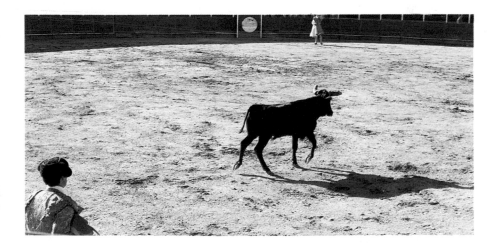

27 The trot in a fighting bull. A symmetrical gait with diagonally opposite limbs used synchronously.

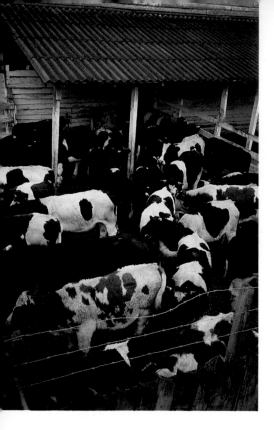

28 Stock should not be mixed at the market if stress and injury are to be minimised (*left*). Isolation and the human presence may also cause stress (*below*).

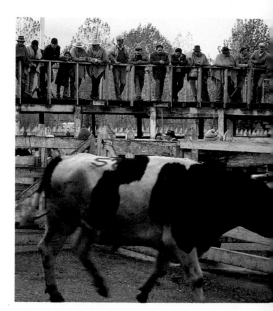

29 Simple hand restraint by positioning the thumb and finger in the nasal orifices, in this case to examine the teeth.

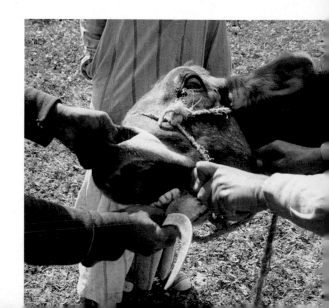

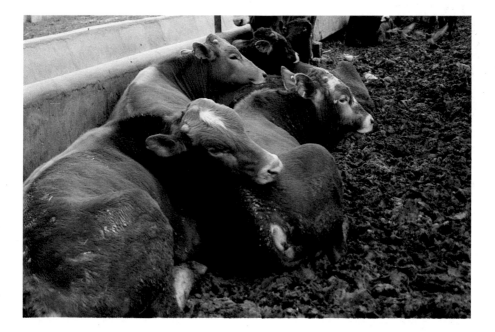

30 Associations during lying.

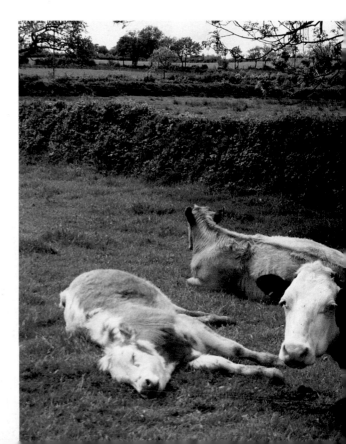

31 Lateral recumbency is most common in young (preruminant) cattle.

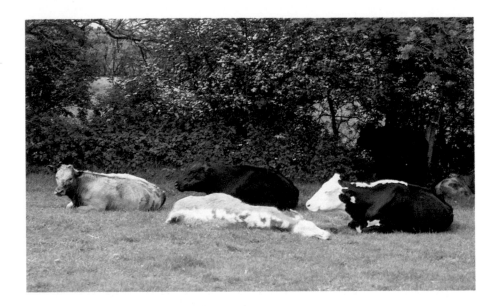

32 Lying is a synchronised activity and cattle often orientate themselves
    in a similar direction. Young cattle especially need protecting and they
    sleep for longer than adult cattle.

33 Cattle do not sleep for long, probably because they evolved without
    secure sleeping sites. Often in a large group one or two 'guard' cattle
    will remain standing while the others lie down.

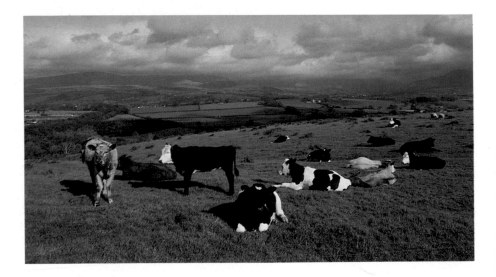

CHAPTER 7

LOCOMOTION AND HANDLING

LOCOMOTION

Locomotion refers to voluntary movements which displace the whole body. This is usually confined to walking, trotting and galloping in cattle, but they can also jump, swim and canter. Other limb movements such as kicking or pawing are performed but do not involve whole body movement.

Locomotion in cattle and indeed all ungulates is primarily by forward motion. Sideways and backward motion *can* be performed but the muscles are designed for forward propulsion, and any other motion is much less efficient. During forward motion the centre of gravity is moved towards the front limb by the propulsive efforts of the hind limb, and the front limb is raised and repositioned to maintain the animal's balance. The positioning of the limbs may be either in a symmetrical or asymmetrical pattern and the animal may be supported by three, two, one or no limbs at any particular time. The faster the gait, the fewer the supporting limbs.

Cattle can only *walk* backwards, and they will do this when confronted with an obstacle in a narrow passageway, such as a race. The same stepping pattern is used as in forward motion and the head is held high to place the centre of gravity as far back as possible.

Cattle change their gait according to their velocity requirements. There is a velocity above which it is energetically more efficient to trot than walk and another where galloping is preferable to trotting.

The Walk

Walking is defined as a gait where each hoof is on the ground for at least 50% of the stride (colour plate 26). The order of hoof movement

151

is shown in Figure 7.1. Each limb is lifted by shortening the leg through flexion of the joints, using especially the hip, knee, hock and digital flexor muscles. The limb then enters the swing phase (Figure 7.2) and is placed on the ground through slow extension of the joint. Once the limb is on the ground, it checks and supports the load by

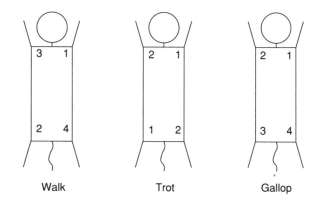

Figure 7.1   Diagrams of cattle gaits. The numbers show the order in which the feet are moved. (Alexander, 1981)

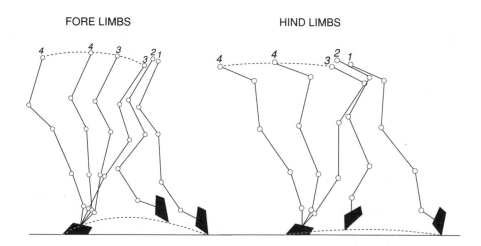

Figure 7.2   Movements of the fore and hind limbs during walking: 1 lifting; 2 swinging; 3 supporting; 4 thrusting. 1 and 2 hanging limb period; 3 and 4 supporting limb period.

tensing all the extensor muscles, particularly in the digital, hock and stifle regions (Nickel *et al.*, 1986). The sole is then pushed hard against the ground by contracting the digital flexors, thus enabling the pushing phase to begin, followed by the hanging limb and swing phases. The limb motion is therefore a cyclical, not an intermittent, process.

The walk can be considered as two people walking out of phase, one behind the other, so that four distinct sounds of the hooves contacting the floor are heard (Figure 7.3). As the walking speed increases, efficiency decreases as the thrust phase (when the limb is supporting) is reduced at the expense of the hanging limb phase (Figure 7.2). The major thrust is provided by the hind legs. The fore limbs, although supporting about 55–60% of the load of the animal, act mainly to position the limbs to enable them to act as support agents and steer the load.

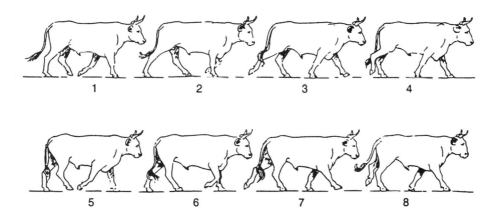

Figure 7.3   Normal walk of the bovine. (Nickel et al., 1986)

During turning the limbs on the outside of the turning circle are abducted or rotated outwards and those on the inside are adducted or rotated inwards (Figure 7.4), resulting in a change in direction. The main pivots for the fore and hind limbs are the shoulder and hip respectively. All limb movements contain an accelerative and a decelerative force. During turning the outer limbs increase their accelerative force while the inner limbs increase their decelerative force. Some abduction and adduction occur during straight walking, but less

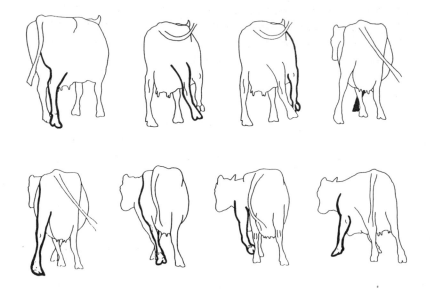

Figure 7.4   Abduction of the outer limb (top) and adduction of the inner limb (bottom) during turning. (Nickel et al., 1986)

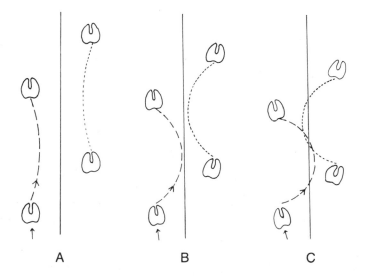

Figure 7.5   Adduction path of the hind limbs of (A) a young non-lactating heifer; (B) a highly bred milking cow; (C) a commonly bred milking cow. (Nickel et al., 1986)

in a well-bred cow or heifer than a badly bred one (Figure 7.5).

Walking behaviour changes with the degree of confidence that cattle have. If the floor is slippery or the building is poorly lit, cattle shorten their stride and slow down the rate of walking.

The Trot

The trot is used by many quadrupeds for long distance motion that is more rapid than the walk. It is a symmetrical gait providing an even motion (colour plate 27). For this reason it is used frequently by cows with full udders, the pendulous nature of which makes the cow reluctant to increase her speed to that of a gallop. When stimulated to move quickly over long periods, as for example if a herdsman hurries a cow down a track for milking, she will trot, as this provides a fast, even motion so that the forces on the udder can be absorbed in a rhythmical swinging motion. In the trot, diagonally opposite limbs are used synchronously: left hind and right front are followed by right hind and left front. In a fast trot there is a period between limb changes when there are no limbs on the ground.

The Gallop

The gallop is the fastest gait and involves an asymmetrical step pattern and a lengthened free-gliding phase. Unlike in smaller mammals, the back in cattle does not contribute to the propulsive force, this being provided mainly by the hind limbs. In the gallop there is a leading front limb, followed by the other front limb, then a pause after which the two hind limbs are placed on the ground, one fractionally before the other.

Motivation for Locomotion

Cattle are motivated to move in response to demand for food, water, companionship, shelter, grooming, a sexual partner, more space and many other resources (Zeeb, 1983). This motivation increases with the duration and severity of resource restriction, especially of space (Dellmeier *et al.*, 1990). It is influenced by many factors, both genotypic and environmental (Figure 7.6).

As animals whose progenitors roamed extensively in search of good grazing, today's cattle appear to need a certain amount of exercise to keep healthy and productive. Regular exercise in the form of supervised walking for tethered cattle will increase muscle and bone growth in growing animals (Melizi, 1985), prevent limb dis-

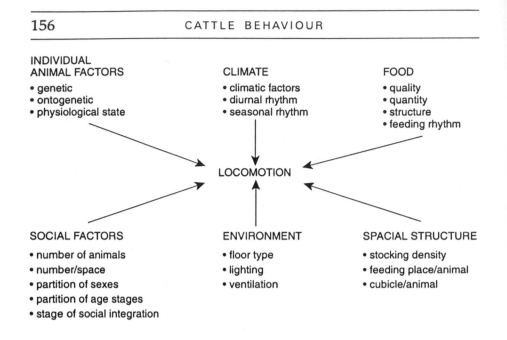

Figure 7.6　Factors influencing cattle locomotion.

orders, especially arthritis in bulls for semen collection, and also improve semen quality in bulls (Vetoshkira, 1985; Zaitser, 1985; and Tizol *et al.*, 1987). Recommended allowances are for about one hour walking per day at about 3–4 km/hour. This recommendation, coupled with the observations that cows in a cubicle house walk for 2–4 km/day (Schofield *et al.*, 1991), suggests that cattle need to walk at least 3 km every day.

Range conditions in Africa may necessitate long-distance walks to water every two or three days. Such travel of up to 40 km to water reduces feed intake and milk production (Homewood *et al.*, 1987; Nicholson, 1989).

Effects of the Environment on Locomotion

The environmental features with the greatest effect on cattle locomotion are the spatial structure and the type of accommodation, including lying and walking areas. These environmental effects undoubtedly interact with each other, and the animal's perception of the environment is modified by its experience.

Space availability

In both housed and grazing cattle the available space is one of the main determinants of locomotory activity. In the grazing situation an increase in area and reduction in food availability forces cattle to walk further to search for food. Cattle on rangeland conditions in the Camargue have been recorded as walking three times as far as cattle on intensively managed pasture (Zeeb, 1983). In intensive grazing the cows only spend a small amount of time each day in between grazing bouts searching for new areas to graze, perhaps ten to twenty minutes.

Increases in locomotion can be caused by external parasites such as flies (Hayakawa, 1984) or bats (Delpietro, 1989), which interrupt grazing activity. This encourages cattle to move about and search for open, windy areas where they can lose the attention of the parasites, which normally attack when the cattle are stationary, especially lying down.

An important consequence of excessive treading activity by cattle on poorly drained and clay soils is the loss of soil stability and eventual poaching damage (Schofield and Hall, 1986) (Plate 7.1).

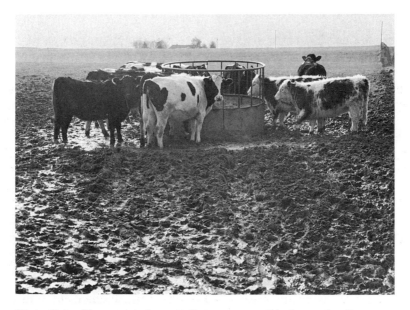

Plate 7.1   Excessive locomotion can result in loss of soil stability and poaching.

With housed cattle the provision of adequate space for locomotion is a complex issue. Although a considerable proportion of locomotion is still associated with feeding, and milking in the case of the dairy cow, a significant amount is associated with social and other activities. This is because cattle eating conserved food spend less time eating than grazing cattle; they are stationary while they eat: and the greater stocking density in a building than at pasture encourages more social interaction, especially grooming.

In a cubicle house for dairy cows the space for walking is provided in the passageways between cubicles, in the feeding passage and sometimes in a separate exercise area (Plate 7.2). If the amount of space provided for locomotion is decreased below 4–5 m²/cow, it is likely that locomotory activity will initially increase for a few days because of aggression caused by competition for space. In the long term, however, locomotion decreases due to the restriction in space availability (Figure 7.7 and Plate 7.3). If an insufficient number of cubicles are provided for lying (Figure 7.8), locomotion increases, particularly in subordinate cows.

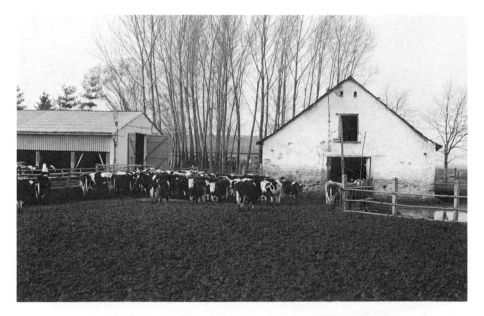

Plate 7.2   Cow accommodation with exercise area. Formerly for tethered cows, this conversion, while providing facilities for locomotory behaviour, does not have a dry lying area in wet weather.

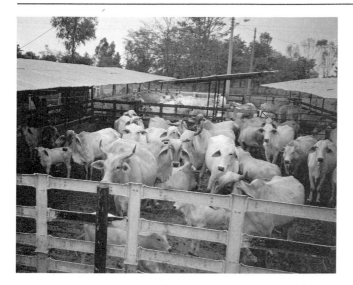

Plate 7.3   Overcrowded cattle show
            reduced locomotion (*above*),
            and injuries which may
            cause lameness are
            common (*right*).

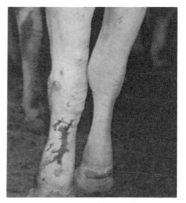

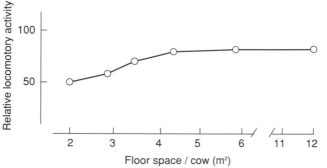

*Figure 7.7   Locomotion changes in relation to space availability. (Zeeb,
1983)*

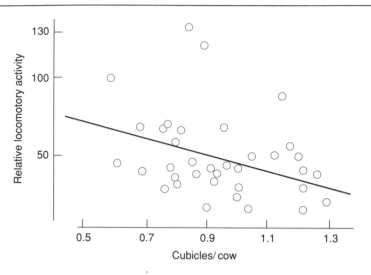

Figure 7.8   Cow locomotion and cubicle availability. (Zeeb and Bammert, 1984)

Floors

The floor is the most important part of the cattle house in its influence on cattle locomotion. Floor properties which influence locomotion include friction, which determines the slipperiness of the floor; hardness, which determines the loading on the limb; and the surface profile, which determines the stress loading on the hoof, as well as interacting with frictional properties of the floor.

Friction can be measured as the force required to start the motion of a cow's hoof across the floor (static friction) or that required to maintain this motion (sliding friction). There are both horizontal and vertical components to this force and the ratio is known as the coefficient of friction. Although it has been found that the number of slip movements by the leg increases rapidly (Figure 7.9) when the coefficient of static friction decreases below 0.4, in practice cattle probably show a consistent increase in floor preference as the coefficient of friction increases (Figure 7.10). If cattle also lie on the floor, as in tie stalls, they may show more injuries to the legs through hairless patches, swellings and wounds and fewer slipping injuries as the coefficient of friction increases.

For loose housing systems where minimising slip is the main concern, the minimum coefficient of friction depends on the surface profile. For solid floors it should be at least 0.4, for slatted floors 0.35

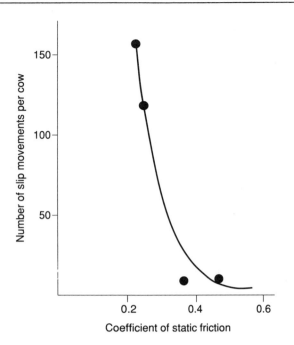

Figure 7.9 Effect of coefficient of static friction on the number of slip movements of four cows during four eating periods. (Webb and Nilsson, 1983)

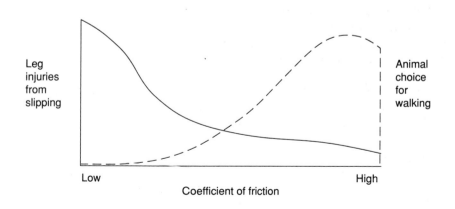

Figure 7.10 Predicted relationship between the coefficient of friction of the floor, the animal choice for walking (– – –) and the number of leg injuries from slipping (————). (Webb and Nilsson, 1983)

and for perforated floors 0.25 (Irps, 1983). The frictional properties of a solid floor may be improved by cutting grooves in a squared pattern with 4 cm sides (Dumelow and Albutt, 1990). This disrupts the floor profile and gives the cow's hoof a greater vertical area against which it can apply pressure during the pushing phase of each stride. Also the repeated passage of cows over a solid floor wears away the deformations in the floor profile created by initial tamping or grooving. Slips in excess of 500 mm are common on slurry-covered smooth concrete, especially during mounting behaviour (Mitchell, 1974). During the slip the hooves, especially in the front feet, turn outwards from the direction of travel.

A comparison of different floor surfaces shows that soil is the most slip resistant, that a covering of slurry increases slip by 56% and that tamping increases slip resistance more than grooving (Table 7.1). On slippery floors cows modify their behaviour to reduce the incidence of slipping. They reduce their speed of walking and reduce the angles of extension of the limbs to the floor (Phillips, 1990). Slip is most likely when the hoof first touches or leaves the floor and the vertical loading is least. The further the hoof is placed in front of or behind the centre of the stride, the less the vertical force and the greater the chance of slip. Hence stride length is reduced as the animal attempts to compensate for the floor conditions.

Slatted floors present a severe obstacle to normal cattle locomotion (Kirchner and Boxberger, 1987). Cattle cannot avoid the slots but their claws often slip into them, causing contusion of the sole and

TABLE 7.1   Slip distances for back feet on different floor surfaces, either dry or covered with slurry.

Surface	Slip (mm)
Dry	
Sandy soil	21
Tamped concrete	29
Grooved concrete	36
Steel float concrete	41
Slurry covered	
Tamped concrete	40
Grooved concrete	54
Steel float concrete	81

(From Albutt *et al.*, 1990)

exungulation. To avoid excessive pressure on the sole, slot width should not exceed 25–30 mm and to prevent faeces building up on the slats each slat should not exceed 80 mm in width. Slats also cause cattle to slip more often and they alter their locomotion posture, orientating their heads more towards the floor (Sommer, 1988).

Light

Light is very important in determining the perception of the environment by cattle. There is a pronounced diurnal rhythm of locomotion (Figure 7.11), with greater activity during daylight hours, especially at sunrise and sunset if the cattle have peak grazing activity at this time or are moving to or from their night resting area. Housed cattle show more activity at night than grazing cattle (Figure 7.12), and reductions in locomotion have sometimes been recorded when a short winter daylength is supplemented with artificial light (Phillips and Schofield, 1989). This may be because aggression between cows (and the consequent increase in locomotion) is reduced. Unexpected encounters are rare when the house is lit, but common in the dark. In less hostile environments for cattle than a highly stocked cubicle house, for example at pasture or in a strawed yard, there is little effect of supplementary light on activity levels. Most cattle seem to prefer a daylength of about 16 hours and naturally have a quiescent period in the early hours of the morning.

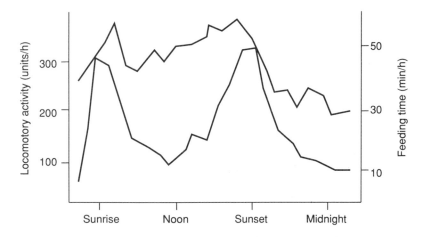

Figure 7.11 Diurnal rhythm of locomotion (top line) and feeding time (bottom line) in Camargue cattle. (Zeeb, 1983)

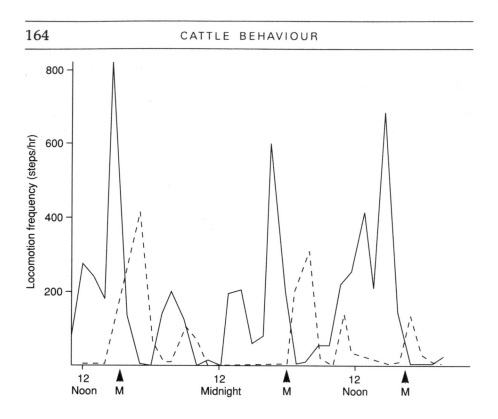

Figure 7.12   Locomotion frequencies of two dairy cows, one active mainly before milking (——) and one active mainly after milking (– – – –), measured with an electric pedometer. (Phillips and Owens, unpublished data)

Animal Factors and Locomotion

Younger cattle, particularly calves at play, are more likely to indulge in the faster forms of locomotion like gambolling and galloping than mature cows, who have little time for such activities and may be hindered from fast movement by the presence of a large udder. Bulls at pasture tend to be more active than cows, especially at night, perhaps because of reduced risk of predation. There is some evidence that hill breeds, such as French Salers cattle, are more active than lowland cattle like the Friesian (Veissier *et al.*, 1989). The introduction of new cattle into a stable group causes increases in activity connected with aggression as the dominance order is sorted out. For instance, the proportion of time spent walking increased from 4% to 6% for three days when ten cows were introduced to a stable group of 50 in a cubicle house (Botto and Zimmermann, 1986).

The oestrous state of cows has a major influence on locomotion, which is typically increased by a factor of 3–4 on the day of oestrus (see Chapter 6). Increased locomotion is also observed just before parturition, whereas it will often decrease after both oestrus and parturition.

Draught Power

A specialised requirement by man involving cattle locomotion is for draught power, where the cattle move not just themselves but also pull a trailed implement or wheeled vehicle (Plate 7.4). Other common forms of work include carrying a load on their back or turning a shaft connected to a power conversion unit, for example to raise water for irrigation (Plate 7.5). The additional load created reduces the speed of locomotion, and cattle increase the thrusting period of the stride (Figure 7.2) and reduce the hanging limb period (Plate 7.6). This also allows some of the energy normally used to decelerate the

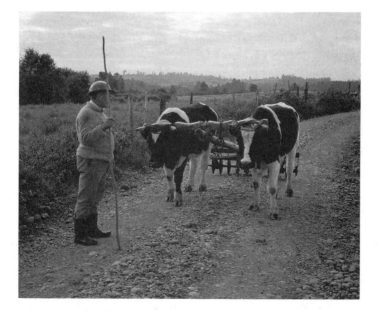

Plate 7.4 Twin yolked bullocks pulling a set of harrowing discs.

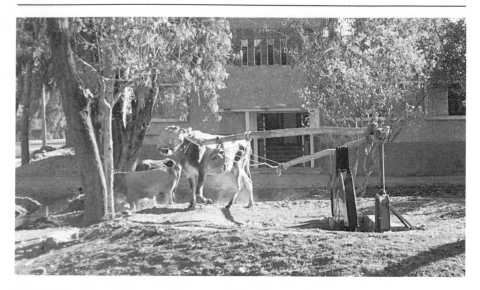

Plate 7.5   Draught power is a specialised form of locomotion. Reducing
the sensory perception by blindfolding encourages locomotion,
probably as an escape response to fear. This is demonstrated
here by a heifer harnessed for raising irrigation water.

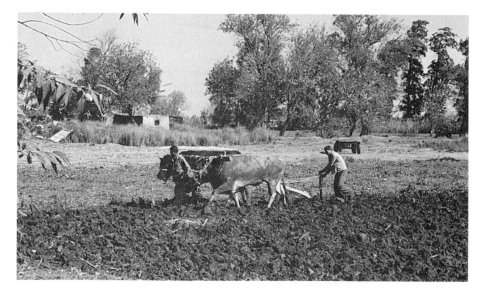

Plate 7.6   During heavy work cattle increase the thrusting period of the
stride and reduce the hanging limb period.

legs to be used for pulling the load. The load is transferred to the animal's shoulders by a collar or a yoke, which may be for one or two animals. The energy cost of the work is related to the ground conditions, the gradient and the type of cattle used. A steady load is easier for cattle to manage than a varying one, and large cattle can cushion variation better than, for example, a donkey.

Cattle prefer to walk at between 0.6 and 1.0 metres/second, and within this 'comfort zone' there is little change in the energetic efficiency of walking (Figure 7.13). If the load is so heavy that the cattle have to pull it very slowly, they behave awkwardly. With heavy loads draught cattle have to use their back as well as their shoulders, and this reduces the energetic efficiency. Above 1 metre/second the energetic efficiency of the work also decreases (Lawrence and Stibbard, 1990). Saddles with loads are borne more efficiently if mounted on the animal's shoulders than its back, because the load is transferred directly to the ground through the front legs, rather than having to stress muscles to dissipate the load.

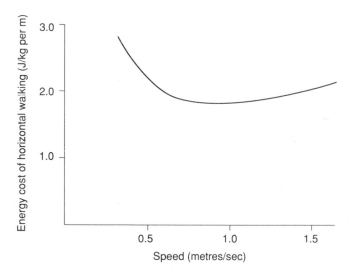

Figure 7.13 *Energy cost of horizontal walking at different speeds. (Ribeiro et al., 1977)*

Lameness

Lameness is the clinical exhibition of an abnormality of the musculoskeletal system in one or more limbs. This abnormality can arise

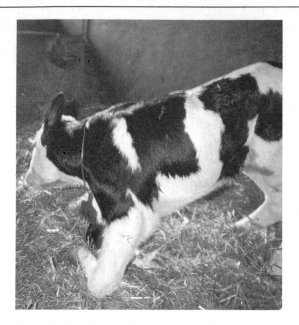

Plate 7.7   Congenital lameness in a young calf.

from many different things: congenital defect, infectious or metabolic diseases, or trauma induced by environmental factors (Plate 7.7). During lameness the supporting or swinging limb periods, or both, are shortened, so that the stride length is reduced. Reduction in the supporting limb period is most common with acutely painful lesions such as a sole abscess or chip fracture, as the pain is accentuated by pressure on the limb. Relief is gained also by relieving pressure on the diseased claw whilst standing (Plate 7.8). When the swinging limb period is contracted this is often associated with increased abduction or adduction as the animals may attempt to decrease load bearing by a particular part of the hoof. Some unevenness of gait is evident before and after each lameness incident, and in total the animal's gait may be affected for three months or more, with the animal being clinically lame on average for about eight weeks (Figure 7.14) (Phillips, 1990). A system of scoring cattle for the severity of lameness, based on the associated behavioural changes, has been devised by Manson and Leaver (Table 7.2). Alternatively, stride length may be measured in lameness research, but there are many sources of variation.

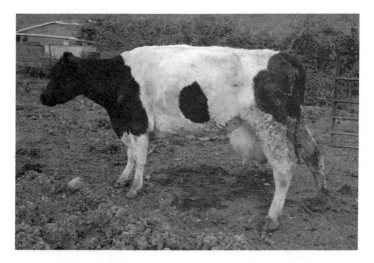

Plate 7.8　Severe lameness in a dairy cow causes loss of body condition. In this case splaying the hind legs reduces the pressure on the diseased outer claw.

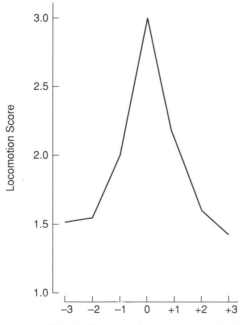

Months before and after lameness incident

Figure 7.14　Change in locomotion score before and after a lameness incident. Locomotion score 1 = even gait with no observable adduction or abduction; 2 = uneven gait but not lame; 3 = lame. (Phillips, 1990)

TABLE 7.2 Description of a locomotion scoring system.

1.0	Minimal abduction/adduction, no unevenness of gait, no tenderness
1.5	Slight abduction/adduction, no unevenness or tenderness
2.0	Abduction/adduction present, uneven gait, perhaps tender
2.5	Abduction/adduction present, uneven gait, tenderness of feet
3.0	Slight lameness, not affecting behaviour
3.5	Obvious lameness, some difficulty in turning, not affecting behaviour pattern
4.0	Obvious lameness, difficulty in turning, behaviour pattern affected
4.5	Some difficulty in rising, difficulty in walking, behaviour pattern affected
5.0	Extreme difficulty in rising, difficulty in walking, adverse effects on behaviour pattern

(Manson and Leaver, 1988)

OTHER FORMS OF MOVEMENT

Apart from locomotion, where the whole animal's body is moved, there are many other limb movements which have a variety of functions. Stretching is one such movement, which affects limb and other muscles. When cattle stretch they tense their muscles in the neck, back and limbs to maintain them in an active state and facilitate blood supply.

Maintaining the muscle tone and exercising the joints is particularly necessary for the foetus since it cannot exercise its limbs by locomotion (Fraser, 1985).

Cattle also use their limbs, particularly the front ones, for manipulation in the same way that we use our hands. They will paw the ground to dig up earth and kick at objects. The limbs are also used to stand up and lie down and to change posture when standing or lying.

BEHAVIOUR DURING HANDLING

Handling Problems

Handling refers to the manipulation and usually the movement of cattle by humans, and usually occurs for the purposes of slaughter, milking, restraint for veterinary work, movement to a different area of the farm on foot or movement in a vehicle to another farm, to market or to an abattoir. Because most cattle are not accustomed to being handled for these purposes, with the exception of milking, stress is likely to result unless the handling procedure is carried out with full regard for the animals' requirements for some continuity of nutritional, social and environmental resources. Their response to handling is highly likely to include abnormal behaviour, which can vary from the mild exhibition of stereotypies to acute distress and even death. Much can yet be done to improve the welfare of cattle during handling, both in refining the environmental and management practices during handling and in developing the handling skills of stock controllers, particularly those operating off the farm, who may have little relevant education or experience. This will have benefits of better labour efficiency and safety, better product quality (especially meat), and enhanced public perception of the cattle production industry.

Handling and Transport to Slaughter

The traditional practice of driving cattle on foot over long distances to slaughter has now largely been superseded by vehicular transport. Previously drovers moved cattle to market at a rate of about 10–15 miles/day and had to protect their stock from excessive hoof wear by shoeing them. Nevertheless the stress on stock was sometimes considerable and losses often high (Chambers and Mingay, 1966).

The most common form of transport to slaughter is by truck. Loading is frequently a stressful procedure, particularly if the angle of the loading ramp is too steep, when cattle are likely to slip. The recommended maximum angle is 20° (Grandin, 1983). Stepped ramps improve the animal's footing (Plate 7.9) and sides are essential. Cattle are also more likely to slip if they are given rough treatment and hurried, especially if electric prods are used. If there is a permanent loading dock, the truck should be positioned so that cattle have no gap to cross. The truck should be loaded from the end so that they do not have to turn a sharp corner as soon as they enter the vehicle. Care should be taken that cattle do not have to move from a poorly lit to a brightly lit area, or vice versa.

Stress in a truck is increased if there are large groups of animals that are unfamiliar with each other, or if the space per animal is insufficient (Table 7.3). If unfamiliar cattle are to be transported in a truck, it is better if they are mixed well before the journey, as otherwise fighting can occur (Connell, 1984).

Once in the truck cattle initially exhibit nervousness, trembling

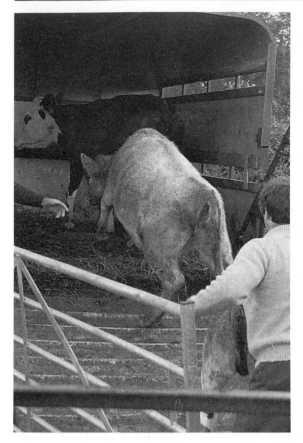

Plate 7.9

Loading cattle into a transport vehicle. A stepped ramp improves the animals' footing.

TABLE 7.3   Recommended space allowances and maximum group size for cattle during road transport.

	Weight (kg)	Space allowance (m²)	Maximum group
Young calves	40–80	0.33	25–30
Old calves	80–150	0.70	15–25
Young steers/heifers	150–300	0.7–1.1	10–15
Older steers	300–700	1.1–1.6	10
Cows	> 450	1.3–1.7	5
Bulls	> 550	1.7–2.0	5

(From Connell, 1984)

and frequent urinating and defecating. After some time, usually between 30 minutes and four hours, they eventually settle and will lie down to rest. During the initial period they stand, most often at right angles to the direction of travel to counteract sideways sway. If possible they will eat and drink, and they often lie down to rest only when the truck is stationary, particularly if the road is rough. Horned cattle are particularly difficult to transport, as they can accidentally injure other stock in moving around. Nevertheless, they should not be tied by the horns, and bulls should not be tied by their rings, or they will be excessively stressed by the constant motion.

Cattle may also be transported by sea, rail or air. A common problem in boats is the failure to provide adequate ventilation, and high temperatures and ammonia accumulation are common. Injuries may also occur due to the rolling action of the ship, but cattle are reputedly more sure-footed than humans in this respect (Collins, 1984). Inadequate attention to pen design and provision of feed and water are frequent problems. Mortality may not always be high during the journey but in calves has been found most likely in the first week after shipment.

Unlike the loading chute, an unloading chute should be wide and straight to give cattle a clear exit route. At the slaughter house or market every effort should be made not to mix stock, particularly bulls, in order that fighting and stress is minimised (colour plate 28). If bulls have to be mixed this is best done after they have been fed. Cattle, especially bulls, should ideally be slaughtered as soon as possible after arrival. Even resting overnight can often lead to carcasses with dark-cutting—a problem associated with pre-slaughter stress.

Races, Crowd Pens and Crushes

Cattle are put into a race either for one-by-one treatment such as drenching, or to move them single file into an area where they can be handled singly, as in a crush or dip. Although they move more easily in the race if it has solid sides, they will accustom to one with open sides, which should preferably be V-shaped to support the animal and prevent them from lying down. Cattle prefer to move in a circular rather than a straight direction (Plate 7.10) (Grandin, 1983), and if they are stressed, bunching may occur. Often an animal may then lie down, and it may be difficult to make it stand again.

In a crowd pen one side is angled at 30° to direct cattle to the entrance of a race. Crowd gates may be used behind the cattle to

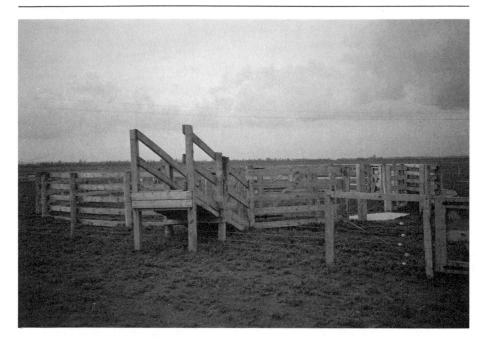

Plate 7.10   A circular cattle handling facility with permanent loading deck.

encourage them to move, but gates should not be electrified nor should electric goads be used or else bunching is likely to occur. Dogs are sometimes used in cattle handling and probably cause less stress than they do to sheep. However, rushing cows down a lane with a dog is not a suitable preparation for milking (Plate 7.11)!

The ideal cattle crush has solid sides to make the animal feel secure, but frequently this is not possible as access is needed, for example to cows' hooves (Plate 7.12). A winch or chain may be used to raise cows' hooves for trimming. A head restraint is useful and usually takes the form of two vertical bars which clamp around the animal's neck. For wild cattle this is not sufficient as vertical movement is still possible. Head restraint can also be achieved by holding the animal's nose with thumb and middle finger in the nostrils (colour plate 29). Bulls often have a permanent ring put in their nose so that they can be led. Other cattle may be led by training them to accept a halter.

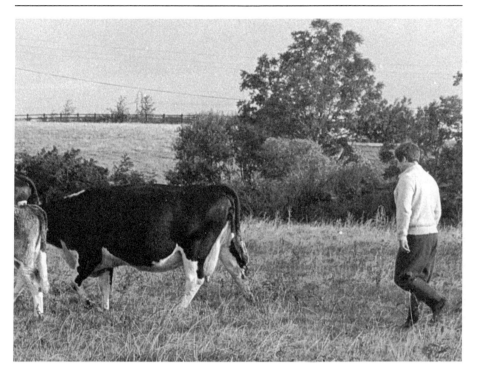

Plate 7.11 Cattle can be moved by a man (*above*) with or without the aid of a horse or dog (*below*).

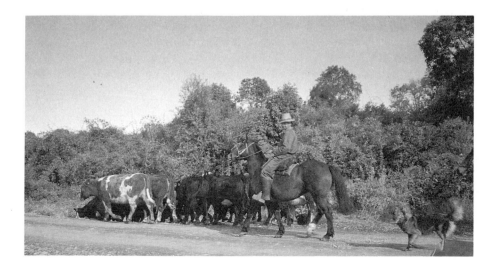

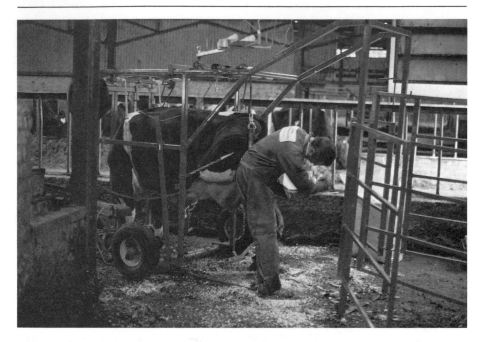

Plate 7.12   An open crush with a winch for hoof trimming.

REFERENCES

Albutt, R. W., Dumelow, J., Cermak, J. P., and Owen, J. E. 1990. 'Slip-resistance of solid concrete floors in cattle buildings.' *Journal of Agricultural Engineering Research*, 45, 137–147.

Alexander, N. 1987. 'Locomotion.' In *The Oxford Companion to Animal Behaviour* (ed. McFarland, D.) pp. 347–356. Oxford University Press, Oxford.

Botto, V., and Zimmermann, V. 1986. 'Effect of group formation on the ethological regime and milk efficiency of cows under conditions of large-scale production.' *Zivocisna-Vyroba*, 31, 983–988.

Chambers, J. D., and Mingay, G. E. 1966. *The Agricultural Revolution, 1750–1880*, pp. 30–33. Batsford, London.

Connell, J. 1984. *International transport of farm animals intended for slaughter*. CEC report EUR 9556 EN. Commission of the European Community, Brussels.

Dellmeier, G., Friend, E., and Gbur, E. 1990. 'Effects of changing housing on open-field behaviour.' *Applied Animal Behaviour Science*, 26, 215–230.

Delpietro, H. A. 1989. 'Case reports on defensive behaviour in equine and bovine subjects in response to vocalisation of the common vampire bat (Desmodus rotundus).' *Applied Animal Behaviour Science*, 22, 377–380.

Dumelow, J. and Albutt, R. 1990. 'The effect of floor design on skid resistance in dairy cattle buildings.' In *Update in Cattle Lameness* (ed. Murray, R.), pp. 130–142. British Cattle Veterinary Association, University of Liverpool.

Fraser, A. F. 1985. Kinetic behaviour of the fetus and newborn. In *Ethology of Farm Animals* (ed. Fraser, A. F.), pp. 111–125. Elsevier, Amsterdam.

Grandin, T. 1983. 'Welfare requirements of handling facilities.' In *Farm Animal Housing and Welfare* (ed. Baxter, S. H., Baxter, M. R., and McCormack, J. A. C.), pp. 137–149. Martinus Nijhoff, The Hague.

Hayakawa, H., Takahashi, H., and Kikuchi, T. 1984. 'Influence of the attack of tabanid flies on the daily behaviour pattern of grazing cattle.' *Annual Report of the Society of Plant Protection of North Japan*, 35, 162–164.

Homewood, K., Rodgers, W. A., and Arhem, K. 1987. 'Ecology of pastoralism in Ngorongoro Conservation Area, Tanzania.' *Journal of Agricultural Science, Cambridge*, 108, 47–72.

Irps, H. 1983. 'Results of research projects into the flooring preference of cattle.' In *Farm Animal Housing and Welfare*, pp. 200–215. Martinus Nijhoff Publishers for CEC. Boston/Den Haag.

Kirchner, M., and Boxberger, J. 1987. 'Loading of the claws and the consequences of the design of slatted floors.' In *Cattle Housing Systems, Lameness and Behaviour*, pp. 37–44. Martinus Nijhoff, Boston/Den Haag.

Lawrence, P. R., and Stibbard, R. J. 1990. 'The energy costs of walking, carrying and pulling loads on flat surfaces by Brahman cattle and swamp buffalo.' *Animal Production*, 50, 29–39.

Manson, F. J., and Leaver, J. D. 1988. 'The influence of concentrate amount on locomotion and clinical lameness in dairy cattle.' *Animal Production*, 47, 185–190.

Melizi, M. 1985. 'Effect of different amounts of forced exercise on patella morphology in young beef bulls. II Morphology of the menisci in cattle in relation to age and exercise.' *Veterinary Bulletin*, Abstract 055, 05334.

Mitchell, C. D. 1974. 'Are the passageways in your cubicle building too slippery?' *Farm Building Progress*, 37, 17–20.

Nicholson, M. J. 1989. 'Depression of dry matter and water intake in Boran cattle, owing to physiological, volumetric and temporal limitations.' *Animal Production*, 49, 29–34.

Nickel, R., Schummer, A., Seiferle, E., Frewein, J., et al. 1986. *The Locomotor System of the Domestic Mammals*. Verlag Paul Parey, Berlin.

Phillips, C. J. C., and Schofield, S. A. 1989. 'The effect of supplementary light on the production and behaviour of dairy cows.' *Animal Production*, 48, 293–303.

Phillips, C. J. C. 1990. 'Pedometric analysis of cattle locomotion.' In *Update in Cattle Lameness* (ed. Murray, R. D.), pp. 163–176. British Cattle Veterinary Association, University of Liverpool.

Riberiro, J. M. de C. R., Brockway, J. M., and Webster, A. J .F. 1977. 'A note on the energy cost of walking.' *Animal Production*, 25, 107–110.

Scholefield, D., and Hall, D. M. 1986. 'A recording penetrometer to measure the strength of soil in relation to the stresses exerted by a walking cow.' *Journal of Soil Science*, 37, 165–176.

Schofield, S. A., Phillips, C. J. C. and Owens, A. R. 1991. 'Variation in the milk production, activity rate and electrical impedance of cervical mucus over the oestrous period of dairy cows.' *Animal Reproduction Science*, 24, 231–248.

Sommer, T. 1985. 'Untersuchungen zur Tiergerchtreit praxisublicher gestaltung von Lauffloechen fur Milchvieh im Boxenlaufstall.' *Liz. Arbect. Zool. Institut.*, Bern.

Tizol, G., Martinez, C., Nunez, E. A., Garcia, H. *et al*. 1987. 'Effect of different levels of exercise on semen quality in Holstein-Friesian bulls.' *Revista de Salud Animal*, 9, 129–137.

Veissier, I., le Neindre, P., and Trillat, G. 1989. 'The use of circadian behaviour to measure adaptation of calves to changes in their environment.' *Applied Animal Behaviour Science*, 22, 1–12.

Vetoshkina, G. A. 1985. 'Effect of exercise on heart in morphometry in cattle II. Effect of age on dimensions of the heart in bulls, in relation to the amount of exercise.' *Veterinary Bulletin*, Abstract 055, 05319.

Webb, N. G., and Nilsson, C. 1983. 'Flooring and injury—an overview.' In *Farm Animal Housing and Welfare*, pp. 226–259. Martinus Nijhoff Publishers for CEC, Boston/Den Haag.

Zaitser, E. A. 1985. 'Preventing hock arthrosis in breeding bulls.' *Veterinary Bulletin*, Abstract 055, 05168.

Zeeb, K. 1983. 'Locomotion and space structure in six cattle units.' In *Farm Animal Housing and Welfare*, pp. 129–136. Martinus Nijhoff Publishers for CEC, Boston/Den Haag.

Zeeb, K., Bock, C., and Heinzler, B. 1983. 'Control of social stress by consideration of suitable space.' In *Social Stress in Domestic Animals* (ed. Zayan, R., and Dantzer, R.), pp. 275–281. Kluwer Academic Publishers, Dordrecht, Netherlands.

Zeeb, K., and Bammert, J. 1984. 'Locomotion and number of cubicles for dairy cows.' In *Proceedings of the 15th International Conference on Angewandite Ethologie bei Nutztierea*. Freiburg, 16 November, 1983.

CHAPTER 8

REST

LYING

Lying is an important behaviour in cattle for which they demonstrate a strong motivation (Metz, 1985). It is used for rest, predator avoidance and association (colour plate 30). Some high-yielding dairy cows need extra rest but have little time available because of the longer periods required for grazing, ruminating, etc. (Venis *et al.*, 1980). In these cows the amount of lying can increase as the lactation progresses and milk yield declines.

A major change in the lying facilities available for housed cows came with the introduction of the cubicle, or free stall. This is a solid bed raised off the floor with partitions to create individual lying areas for the cows. If the cubicle bed is too small, which is increasingly common with the greater size of the modern dairy cow, the cow will have difficulty lying down or getting up (Plate 8.1). This leads to swellings on the hocks or the knees and encourages cows to be either half in the cubicle or in the passageway (Plate 8.2). Some improvements in the use of cubicles can be achieved by training calves and heifers to accept a smaller version of the cubicle (Plate 8.3).

The amount of lying averages 13 hours/day for calves (Weiguo and Phillips, 1991), 12 hours/day for bulls (Houpt and Wollney, 1989) and 7–10 hours/day for lactating dairy cows (in approximately 5 periods of 1.5 hours each) (Arave and Walters, 1980).

When a cow lies down in a cubicle she normally kneels down with one foreleg, then both, and then tucks one hind limb under her abdomen as she lowers her rear end (Figure 8.1). Thus when lying down the cow eases her centre of gravity forwards along a longitudual axis to minimise the stress on the limbs. Adequate space for

179

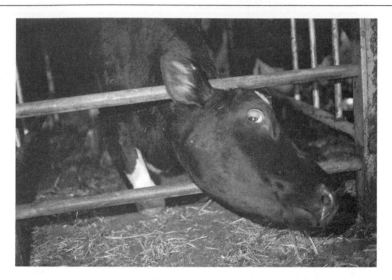

Plate 8.1   Difficulties in manoeuvring in a cubicle because of inadequate lunging space.

Plate 8.2   Cubicle rejection. Cows lying in the passageway become dirty and are likely to have their teats trodden on by other cows.

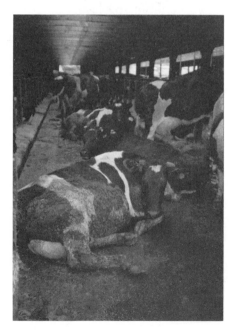

Plate 8.3   A calf learning to use a cubicle.

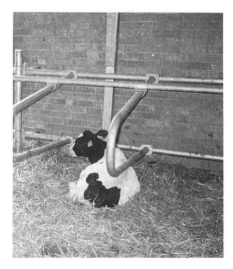

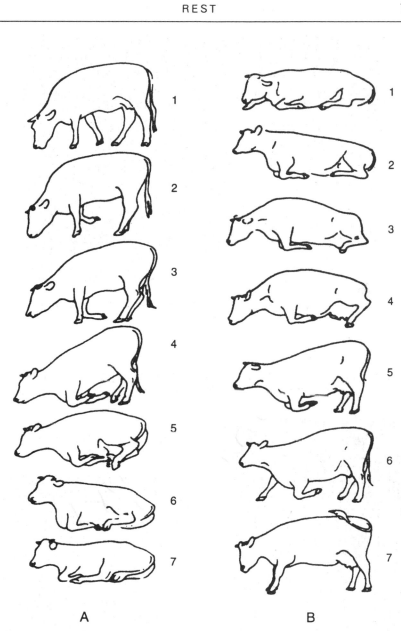

Figure 8.1   The sequence of lying (A) and standing (B). (Fraser and Broom, 1990)

forward motion is essential for cow comfort, both when lying down and when rising (Figure 8.2). When rising, the cow first raises her fore quarters slightly and then her hind quarters, using the outer hind leg primarily for vertical propulsion, then the inner hind leg that was tucked under, the fore leg on the same side and finally the outer front leg (Figure 8.1).

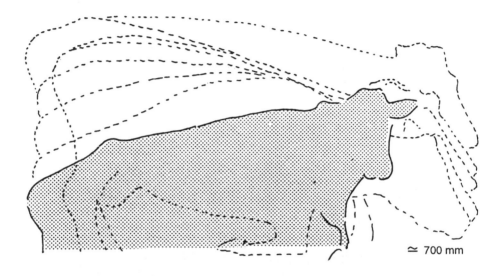

Figure 8.2   Forward space demand of rising movement (800 kg Friesian cow). (Cermak, 1987)

Pregnant cows often prefer to lie on their left side, probably because the foetus dwells in the right side of the abdominal cavity, at least in the latter stages of pregnancy. On average about one-third of cows show a clear preference for right- or left-side laterality. As the cows get older they show less preference for left-side laterality, possibly because there is more room in the abdominal cavity and less chance of damage to the foetus by lying on the right side (Arave and Walters, 1980). If there is a slope on the cubicle the cows prefer to lie with their dorsal side uphill. If a cubicle to one side is occupied, a cow prefers to lie with her back next to the cow's back in the adjoining cubicle. If cubicles are positioned end to end with open fronts, as is sometimes advocated to allow adequate lunging space, the cows are reluctant to lie facing each other. In fact they seem to prefer a cubicle with a solid front, which does limit lunging space but gives greater comfort and a feeling of enclosed personal space.

Most adult cattle lie in the sternally recumbent position, that is, on the sternum or breast bone. Occasionally they will lie laterally recumbent (flat out) although not generally in cubicles because of restricted space. Prolonged lateral recumbency is prevented by the need to eructate gases from the rumen at regular intervals (Plate 8.4). Gravity plays an important part in reticulo-ruminal function and in releasing the gas bubble (normally present in the dorsal sac of the rumen) to the atmosphere via the oesophagous (Balch, 1955). Calves without a fully developed rumen often lie for sometime in the laterally recumbent position (colour plate 31). Beef cattle that are very fat occasionally have difficulty in maintaining a sternally recumbent position and may roll over onto their side.

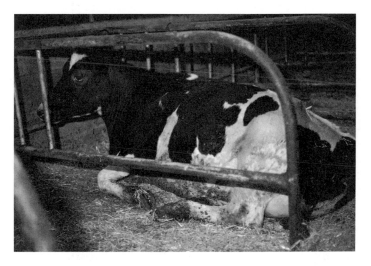

Plate 8.4   The cubicle prevents the cow from adopting
a laterally recumbent position.

Cubicles

There are many different types of cubicle division available (Figure 8.3), all attempting to effectively separate the cows while minimising

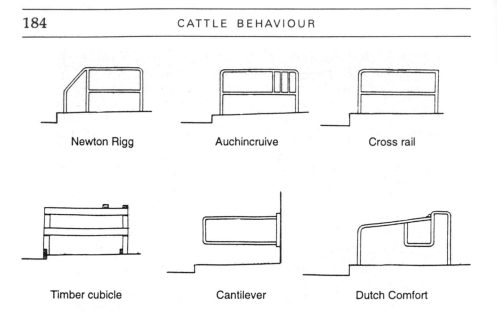

Newton Rigg   Auchincruive   Cross rail

Timber cubicle   Cantilever   Dutch Comfort

Figure 8.3   Some cubicle divisions for dairy cows. (Loynes, 1985)

the hindrance to the cows' movements caused by the hardware (Plate 8.5). A modern design that allows some space-sharing by virtue of the absence of a bottom rail at the back of the cubicle is the Dutch Comfort design. If there is a bottom rail it should be about 50 cm from the cubicle base to avoid cows becoming trapped underneath. Front rails, which prevent the cow moving too far into the cubicle and becoming trapped, should be either near the floor (<25 cm from the floor) or on the top rail; otherwise the rail will impede a cow's rising. In Dutch Comfort cubicles the front hoop should not be wider than 35 cm or small cows can get their shoulders stuck. Some cubicles should always be able to accommodate the largest cows in the herd.

Cubicle length can be worked out using the cow's weight: length (m) equals $1.75 + 0.00068 \times$ weight (kg) (Cermak, 1987), and the width is usually half the length. A variety of bedding materials can be used to increase cow comfort, especially when lying down, and also to absorb any urine deposited in the cubicle. A neck rail can be positioned perpendicular to the divisions, attached to the top rail 45 cm from the wall. This forces the cow to reverse out of the cubicle as she stands up and prevents the bedding being soiled. If cows are not able to stand fully in the cubicle, they will often stand half in and

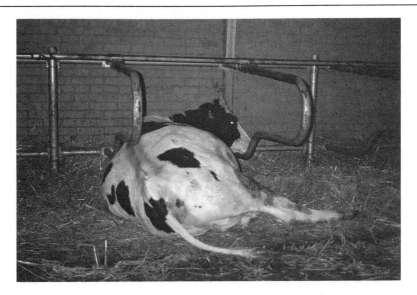

Plate 8.5   A modern cubicle design that allows space-sharing
by virtue of its simple, unrestricting design.

half out, which may increase stress to the hind feet. This is common
in subordinate cows, who use the cubicle as a place of escape.

Bedding material on the cubicle base should be sufficient to
cushion the shock to the cow's limbs as she lies down. It should also
have insulatory properties for young calves kept in low temperatures. The lower critical temperature can increase from 8°C for a calf
on dry straw to 17°C for the same calf on dry concrete. When the
temperature falls outdoors, cattle lie down for longer so as to reduce
heat loss from the underside of the body.

Tethering cattle restricts their lying, at least for the first few weeks,
when they display more intention of lying but fewer actual bouts of
lying, and when stress levels are increased (Ladewig and Smidt,
1989) (Plate 8.6).

SLEEP

Sleep is characterised by a temporary period of inactivity and a
raised response threshold. It is exhibited in a distinct diurnal rhythm

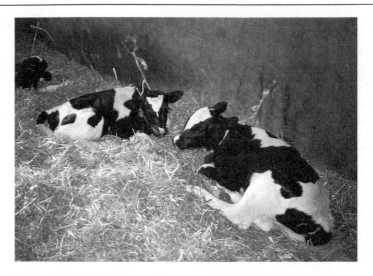

Plate 8.6   Tethering cattle can restrict their lying and
             other behaviour, in this case preventing lateral
             recumbency and posture changes.

and with a characteristic posture. In cattle this is usually in the
sternally recumbent position with the head either resting on the
ground or tucked round and held against the thorax (Plate 8.7).

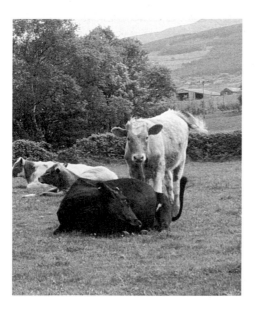

Plate 8.7   Characteristic sleep
             position in cattle, with
             head tucked round
             against the thorax.

Four levels of alertness can be distinguished in cattle (Ruckebush, 1972):

- Alert wakefulness (AW)   Eyes fully open, characterised by a low voltage, fast-activity electroencephalographic (EEG) output by the brain.
- Drowsiness (DR)   Upper eyelid relaxed, increased arousal threshold and reduced alertness. Some high voltage, slow-activity EEG output.
- Quiet sleep (QS)   Eyes almost closed, increased arousal threshold and all EEG output of the high voltage, slow-activity type.
- Active sleep (AS)   Eyes fully closed, all EEG output of the low voltage, fast-activity type, some rapid eye movement (REM), heightened arousal threshold. Otherwise known as paradoxical sleep.

The different proportions of the day spent in the different states are shown in Table 8.1. AW tends to predominate during the day and DR at night. AS only occurs at night and often after a bout of rumination. Rumination often accompanies DR at night and also may accompany AW and occasionally QS. QS in many animals is preceded by regular monotonous actions like ruminating. Reticuloruminal motility is decreased at night, probably because of reduced basal metabolic rate during DR and QS.

The normal transition is from AW to DR to QS to AS. Periods of AS are short in cattle in comparison with other mammals, typically only five minutes long, but they are numerous, usually about ten occurring each night. Hence sleep in cattle can be considered as polyphasic in contrast to humans. Sleep is also characterised by its consistency, as patterns vary little from day to day but are specific to individuals. Occasionally during AS, cattle demonstrate tachycardia,

TABLE 8.1   Proportions of the 24-hour day and of the night spent in alert wakefulness (AW), drowsiness (DR), quiet sleep (QS) and active sleep (AS).

	AW	DR	QS	AS
% of 24 hours	52	31	13	3
% of night	16	52	26	6

(From Ruckebush, 1972)

rapid breathing and/or limb movements which are indicative of dreaming. This phenomenon is not as common as in other ungulates and is most likely to occur in juveniles. The amount of both AS and QS declines with age, and the proportion of sleep that is AS declines from almost 100% at birth to 25% at maturity (Ellingson, 1972).

Functions of Sleep

There are two probable functions of sleep: immobilisation and recuperation (Webb, 1979) (colour plate 32). In some animals regular temporary immobilisation is beneficial in guarding against predation, providing that the sleeping site is secure. In large grazing prey animals this is often not the case, and hence most grazing ungulates have short sleep periods (Meddis, 1975, 1987) (colour plate 33). In contrast for most forest-dwelling prey such as the dormouse, safe sleeping sites are available and sleeping times are long, even extending to hibernation in many species. Thus immobilisation offers two evolutionary advantages—energy conservation, which is of use to predator and prey alike, and security from predation since most predators search for moving prey.

Recuperation is likely to be of some (but perhaps not major) importance, since prolonged deprivation leads to a state of exhaustion, the exhibition of abnormal behaviours and even hysterias. However, there is no evidence that longer sleep patterns occur more frequently in 'higher' animals, suggesting that recuperation of brain function is not important. Indeed AS may specifically function to maintain the brain in a state of readiness during the subconscious state. Also animals that are physically more active do not use sleep more as a method of recuperation. On the contrary many inactive or sporadically active animals such as sloths, bears and lions sleep for long portions of the day. It appears that the choice of whether to become an active feeder for most of the day and minimise sleep, or whether to save energy by minimising sleep, is determined by the security of the sleeping site and the rate at which the ingested food can be digested. Cattle evolved the rumination process to be able to survive on an otherwise relatively indigestible food, but to achieve this they had to sacrifice many hours that could have been spent sleeping. Rumination only rarely accompanies QS and never AS. Hence the proportion of time spent in DR is much higher than in most other animals. Some reduction of basal metabolic rate is achieved but not as much as in QS.

REFERENCES

Arave, C. W., and Walters, J. L. 1980. 'Factors affecting lying behaviour and stall utilisation of dairy cattle.' *Applied Animal Ethology*, 6, 369–376.

Balch, C. C. 1955. 'Sleep in ruminants.' *Nature*, 175, 940–941.

Cermak, J. 1987. 'The design of cubicles for British Friesian dairy cows with reference to body weight and dimensions, spatial behaviour and upper leg lameness.' In *Cattle Housing Systems, Lameness and Behaviour*, (ed. Wierenga, H. K., and Peterse, D. J.), pp. 119–128. Martinus Nijhoff, Dordrecht.

Ellingson, R. J. 1972. Development of wakefulness-sleep cycles and associated EEG patterns in mammals. In *Sleep and the Maturing Nervous System*, (ed. Clemente, C. D., Purpura, D. P., and Mayer, F. E.), pp. 165–174. Academic Press, New York.

Fraser, A. F., and Broom, D. M. 1990. *Farm Animal Behaviour and Welfare.* Baillière Tindall, London.

Houpt, K. A., and Wollney, G. 1989. 'Frequency of masturbation and time budgets of dairy bulls used for semen production.' *Applied Animal Behaviour Science*, 24, 217–225.

Ladewig, J., and Smidt, D. 1989. 'Behaviour, episodic secretion of cortisol and adrenocortical reactivity in bulls subjected to tethering.' *Hormones and Behaviour*, 23, 344–360.

Loynes, I. F., 1985. 'Dairy buildings—where now?' *Farm Buildings Association Journal*, 34, 39–41.

Meddis, R. 1975. 'On the function of sleep.' *Animal Behaviour*, 23, 676–691.

Meddis, R. 1987. 'Sleep.' In *The Oxford Companion to Animal Behaviour* (ed. McFarland, D.), pp. 512–517. Oxford University Press, Oxford.

Metz, J. 1985. 'The reaction of cows to a short-term deprivation of lying.' *Applied Animal Behaviour Science*, 13, 301–307.

Ruckebush, Y. 1972. 'The relevance of drowsiness in the circadian cycle of farm animals.' *Animal Behaviour*, 20, 637–643.

Venis, J., Bajnar, Z., and Navratil, J. 1980. 'Daily behaviour of dairy cows in groups of different size and at different stages of lactation under conditions of free housing in a large cowshed with cubicles.' *Dairy Science Abstracts 1984*, 046-00258.

Webb, W. B. 1979. 'Theories of sleep functions and some clinical functions.' In *The Functions of Sleep* (ed. Drucker, C. R., Shkurovich, M., and Sterman, M. B.), pp. 19–35. Academic Press, New York.

Weiguo, L., and Phillips, C. J. C. 1991. 'The effects of supplementary light on the behaviour and performance of calves.' *Applied Animal Behaviour Science*, 30, 27–34.

CHAPTER 9

BEHAVIOURAL ADAPTATION TO INADEQUATE ENVIRONMENTS

BEHAVIOURAL NEEDS

Keeping cattle in intensive environments inevitably leads to a modification of their behaviour compared with wild cattle. There are, in fact, no wild cattle with which we can compare their behaviour, as the last members of the aurochs or wild cattle (*Bos primigenius*) were killed by poachers on a hunting reserve near Warsaw, Poland in 1627 (Felius, 1985). However, the behaviour of domestic cattle reintroduced into wild or semi-wild environments has been quite regularly observed (e.g. Reinhardt and Reinhardt, 1981). This gives us some idea of what is 'normal' behaviour for the subspecies, although it can be argued that domestication has modified their behaviour sufficiently to make a consideration of behaviour in the wild irrelevant. Nevertheless it is now accepted that farm animals have certain behavioural needs, if not rights, and one of these is to be able to express most normal patterns of behaviour (Webster *et al.*, 1986). Other needs relate mainly to the avoidance of adverse conditions: freedom from thirst, hunger, malnutrition, prolonged discomfort, injury, disease, fear and stress (Webster, 1987).

Behavioural needs are better determined by first investigating, what the innate behaviours are that cattle need to perform, and second what behaviours are required to meet their physiological needs. Physiological needs include the absorption of adequate nutrient supply from the gastrointestinal tract, the perpetuation of the genotype by reproduction and the adequacy of the environment in terms of thermal and other sensory requirements. Taking these into account the major behavioural needs can be categorised as follows:

- Reaction to danger (flight and escape)

- Ingestion
- Body care (including elimination)
- Motion
- Exploration/territorialism
- Rest
- Association (including socialisation and coitus)

Within this framework it must be recognised that all animals, and particularly domesticated animals, are to some extent behaviourally elastic, i.e. they can modify their behaviour to meet their physiological needs. For instance, when a grass sward declines in height, cattle graze for longer and bite faster to try to maintain their intake (see page 83). The extent of this behavioural elasticity is frequently not known and this is one reason why observation of wild cattle may not help in determining the behavioural adequacy of intensive cattle husbandry systems. It can be measured to some extent by depriving cattle of the opportunity to express two or more major behaviours. After the period of deprivation the cattle are observed to see which behaviour they perform. Alternatively, lever-pressing experiments in which cattle are made to work in order to be allowed to perform a certain behaviour can be employed (see pages 21–22).

It seems likely that behavioural elasticity is limited with regard to innate behaviours in the neonate. In calves a particularly innate neonatal motivation is that of suckling. Preventing a calf from performing natural suckling behaviour is known to result in behavioural problems such as sucking the pen or nearest neighbour (kissing). These behavioural problems are relatively well researched in cattle. In the past many people referred to them as 'vices', but as this implies that it is the cattle and not the system that are at fault, it is an unfortunate term to use. 'Abnormal' behaviours are also referred to (see, for example, Wiepkema *et al.*, 1983) but are difficult to define unless we know exactly what is meant by normal behaviour.

Behavioural problems are difficult to categorise, as each one has its own aetiology and function. However, we may discern the following major types, which are not mutually exclusive: stereotyped behaviours, injurious behaviours and redirected behaviours. These may create problems for either the animals, especially injurious behaviours, or the production system in which they are kept, e.g. feed tossing (see page 88) or dark-cutting, which is common in bulls that have fought before slaughter. In addition there are numerous examples of behavioural elasticity or accommodation which are not always deleterious to the animals or the farming system, e.g. abnormal styles of lying or standing, locomotion or nutritional modification.

BEHAVIOURAL PROBLEMS

Stereotyped Behaviours

In many situations cattle exhibit frequent repeated sequences of activity, which are stereotyped. These may be part of the normal behaviour, e.g. grazing or rumination, but in inadequate environments specific repeated sequences of movement may develop which appear to have no direct purpose. These are performed at more than the normal incidence and reoccur in nearly the same order in successive cycles. In cattle they are seen particularly in intensive housing situations and often relate to oral behaviours, such as tongue rolling, bar biting, etc. In tongue rolling the tongue is wrapped around an imaginary tuft of grass, with the head in the upright position (Plate 9.1). It may be a form of redirected sward grasping behaviour as it is not observed in herbivores that bite rather than grasp and tear the sward as cattle do. As discussed with feed tossing behaviour, which may conceivably be redirected sward tearing behaviour, sward grasping behaviour would normally be performed 30,000–40,000 times/day by grazing cattle.

Plate 9.1   Tongue-rolling, probably a redirected grazing activity. (H. H. Sambraus)

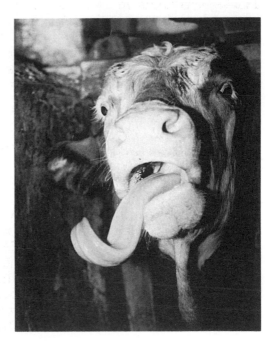

Non-nutritive sucking is common in calves where the sucking motivation is thwarted by supplying milk in a bucket rather than through a teat. Many modern systems now recognise this need and provide milk through a teat, even if it is only floating in the bucket! The satiation of the sucking motivation may otherwise be achieved by sucking the bars in the pen, the bucket handles or any other suitable protrusions. It also encourages calves to suck each other, either by oral 'kissing' or sucking ears and navels. This can lead to transfer of diseases and can be maintained into adulthood in the form of cows sucking each other's teats (and obtaining a further nutritive reward) or prepuce sucking (Plate 9.2) and urine drinking in bulls. The importance of the sucking motivation has been demonstrated by Hammell *et al.* (1988), who showed that providing

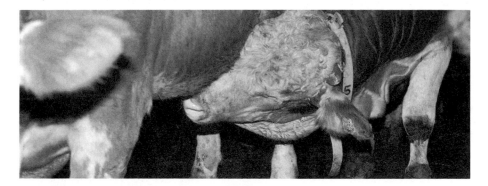

Plate 9.2   Prepuce sucking in bulls. The sucker reaches under a bull (*above*) and stimulates it to urinate (*below*) by licking the prepuce. (H. H. Sambraus)

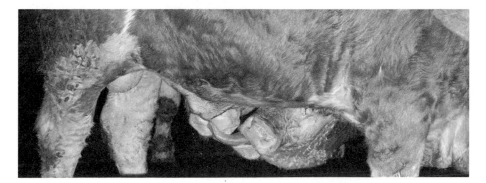

a dummy teat to bucket-fed calves partially satiates the motivation, which is particularly strong at feeding times.

One of the functions of stereotyped behaviours, or stereotypies as they are sometimes known, is to reduce the response threshold and pacify the animal to allow it to cope with a barren environment. In fact drowsiness is common in cattle during the prolonged periods of rumination, and this may be one reason why stereotyped behaviours are less common in ruminant cattle in intensive environments than in other captive animals in intensive environments.

Stereotypies are most likely to occur where there is a specific releaser as well as a predisposing early experience of learning behavioural abnormalities. A common releaser is the lack of fibrous food, which has been linked to sham chewing in veal calves and tongue rolling in bulls. Inadequacy of water supply may trigger prepuce sucking and urine drinking in bulls and milk drinking in cows (Sambraus and Gotthardt, 1985). In such cases these abnormal behaviours may develop in the majority of the animals and may occupy several hours each day.

That these stereotypies perform a useful function in helping animals to cope with an inadequate environment is indisputable. Animals that do not learn to perform these behaviours frequently develop clinical disease problems, such as ulcers (Wiepkema et al., 1987). In this respect stereotypies should be considered as indicators of an inadequate environment, not necessarily as behavioural problems in their own right. This does not necessarily mean that we should attempt to change all husbandry systems where stereotypies are displayed. Humans also exhibit a great deal of stereotyped behaviour in environments that do not cater for all their needs, and they should perhaps have a higher priority for environmental modification. Nevertheless, where the incidence of stereotypies is widespread and lasts for a significant part of the day, this is an indication that the animal is having to devote considerable effort in coping with its environment and modifying it could improve the productive efficiency as well as the welfare of the animal.

That stereotypies are learnt and not innate is apparent because they tend to increase with age. This increase is probably associated with the positive feedback of sensory stimulation and possibly a progressive desensitisation of the repeatedly activated neural systems (Dantzer, 1986). The activation of neural systems has been demonstrated by administering psychostimulants, such as apomorphine (Sharman and Stephens, 1974). These block the neurotransmitters in the brain and cause stereotypies to be performed. In stressed cattle, particularly those suffering from inadequate space or nutrition, it is likely that the release of endogenous brain opioid peptides induces analgesia or a raised pain threshold. This compensates for the lack of arousal and helps the animal to cope with the environment (Dantzer, 1986).

Injurious Behaviours

Behaviours that cause injury to other animals are most common where animals are group housed in a deficient environment. Bulls in a slatted floor building are one example of this, and deleterious behaviours such as excessive mounting (Plate 9.3) and prepuce sucking will often develop. However, injurious behaviours in cattle are not as damaging as in pigs and poultry where the degree of intraspecific aggression may even lead to cannabalism. This may be because of the more gregarious nature of ruminants, and a greater ability to tolerate the close proximity of herdmates, or it may be because of the natural pacifying effect of rumination.

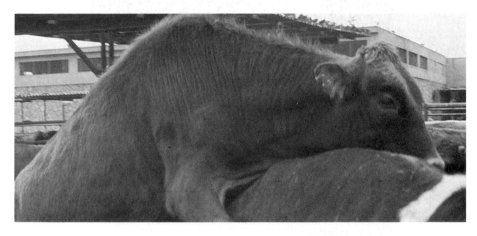

Plate 9.3   The buller steer syndrome. Excessive mounting by steers can lead to exhaustion and slow growth.

Cattle may also indulge in behaviours that are injurious to themselves, such as excessive self-grooming by individually penned calves which can lead to the formation of hairballs in the stomach. Indeed, behaviours during stress often involve excessive toilet activity, particularly self-grooming if cattle are penned and allo-grooming if they are in groups. The use of the tether, which prevents this important stress-dissipating behaviour from taking place, is now increasingly seen as unacceptable on welfare grounds. The process of adaptation to tethering includes initial escape attempts, followed by 'learned helplessness' which is accompanied by extreme passiveness, then the exhibition of stereotyped behaviours (Plate 9.4). These are initially directed to the environment but may increasingly involve self-attention as time progresses.

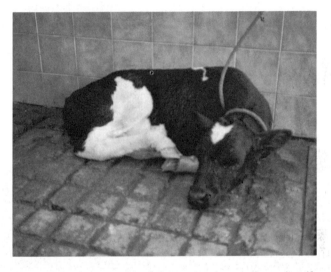

Plate 9.4 Learned helplessness in a tethered calf.

Redirected Behaviours

Where the motivation for a behavioural need is particularly strong and is thwarted by environmental insufficiency, animals may attempt to redirect the motivation to the performance of a similar behaviour. This is especially common with ingestion.

An abnormal diet will often precipitate abnormal oral behaviours, and deficiencies of fibre, phosphorus and sodium will produce cravings for the nutrient, or pica. These may be satiated by unnatural food objects such as wood for fibre, bones for phosphorus and urine for sodium. Cattle that are deficient in sodium often induce urination by prepuce sucking (Stephens, 1974).

Although locomotory activity is common in free-ranging calves, including running, gambling, cantering, as well as many other movements like kicking, jumping etc, the use of redirected behaviours to overcome the restriction of activity in penned calves is limited (Plate 9.5). In other mature stock, behaviours such as weaving, pacing and rocking from one leg to the other are used but in calves these are not commonly seen. Probably these behaviours do not have time to develop in the short period during which dairy calves are penned, and in veal calves other deficiencies such as fibre cause redirected oral behaviours to predominate.

WELFARE

The term 'welfare' is used in a variety of contexts and with a variety of meanings (see Kilgour and Dalton, 1984). Scientists often consider it as the 'animal's state with regard to its attempts to cope with its environment' (Broom, 1986). It is important to remember that internal psychological factors will greatly influence an animal's success in 'coping' with life. Early experience will also have a profound influence—an animal may learn to cope with an inadequate environment by gradually adjusting to increasing stress levels.

In reality there is the element of human perception: two people may agree about the conditions in which an animal is kept and even about the animal's success in coping with the conditions but may profoundly disagree about whether the welfare is good or not. In this context, welfare is best considered as the human perception of the quality of life that an animal has, particularly in relation to its success in coping with its environment.

The transition from good to bad welfare is illustrated in Figure 9.1. As the animal passes from a good to a worse environment it moves from a state of harmony, or equilibrium, to one where it recognises an environmental deterioration. This can be detected experimentally by preference tests, indicating which environment the animal prefers. These must be treated with caution for several reasons: animals may give an exaggerated or diminished response according to previous experience, they may not be sufficiently experienced to choose the best environment for themselves in the long term and their immediate reaction may differ substantially from their long-term one if they are attracted by the novelty of one or more of the environments.

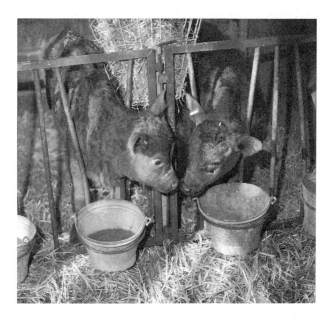

Plate 9.5   Traditional calf rearing systems limit contact with other calves and force the calf to drink unnaturally from a bucket (*above*). Modern systems (*below*) allow for group rearing and teat feeding.

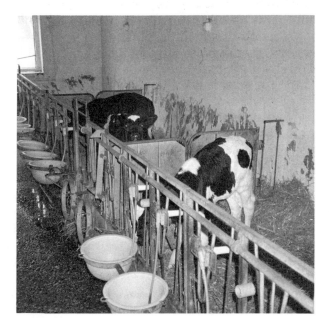

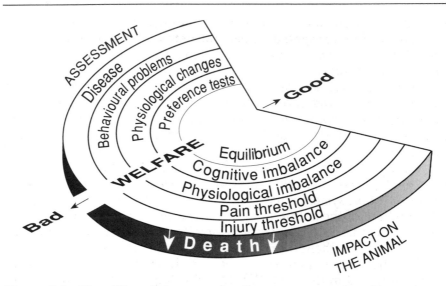

Figure 9.1   *The different degrees of welfare, assessment and impact on the animal.*

A cognitive imbalance may turn into a physiological imbalance if the environment progressively deteriorates. Later pain may be felt and injuries sustained, both of which will tend to cause abnormal behaviour. Disease may follow and may result ultimately in death of the animal.

THE DOMESTIC CONTRACT

By keeping domestic animals in confined conditions, man clearly reduces the freedom of the animal to perform certain desirable behaviours. It may not be essential that these behaviours are performed exactly as they would be in the wild, e.g. some reduction in locomotion can be accepted, and copulation can be replaced by artificial control by humans. However, if we are to demonstrate a healthy respect for the needs of other species with which we share the environment (which has been the hallmark of most successful and sustainable societies to date), we must recognise that the removal of the freedom to perform certain behaviours must be compensated by other provisions. Where we take away on the one hand freedom for locomotion, freedom to copulate and freedom to ingest feeds in a natural manner, we must compensate by, for example, providing freedom to develop bonds with similar livestock, freedom from predation and freedom to ingest adequate nutrients. This may be seen as the formation of a domestic contract that demonstrates our respect for our husbanded livestock.

This respect was an essential feature of most primitive societies, and still is of many modern ones. In many ancient civilisations (Plate 9.6), this respect even went as far as the deification or sanctification of cattle, because of the dependence that man had on them as the major meat and milk producer. However, in the Western world many people are now far removed from the cattle that provide food for them and may through ignorance and/or greed encourage intensive production systems that provide cheap products at the expense of the welfare of the animals in these systems. A better knowledge of cattle behavioural requirements by stockmen, farmers and researchers should enable them to be kept in a manner in which we can truly say that they have enjoyed as good facilities and lifestyle as they would have had in the wild. Whether this happens or not will be for every civilised society to determine.

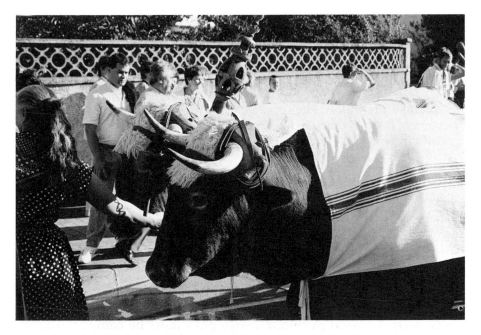

Plate 9.6 Man's dependence on cattle has often led to their being given a sacred status in society. Here cattle are paraded in France adorned with ceremonial white robes and a sceptre.

REFERENCES

Broom, D. M. 1986. 'Indicators of poor welfare.' *British Veterinary Journal*, 142, 524–526.

Dantzer, R. 1986. 'Behavioural, physiological and functional aspects of stereotyped behaviour: a review and a reinterpretation.' *Journal of Animal Science*, 62, 1776–1786.

Felius, M. 1985. 'Genus Bos: Cattle breeds of the world'. p. ix. MSD Agvet, Rahway, New Jersey.

Hammell, K. L., Metz, J. H. M., and Mekking, P. 1988. 'Sucking behaviour of dairy calves fed milk ad libitum by bucket or teat.' *Applied Animal Behaviour Science*, 20, 275–285.

Kilgour, R., and Dalton, C. 1984. *Livestock Behaviour—a Practical Guide*, pp. 281–282. Granada, London.

Reinhardt, V., and Reinhardt, A. 1981. 'Cohesive relationships in a cattle herd (Bos indicus).' *Behaviour*, 77, 121–151.

Sambraus, H. H., and Gotthardt, A. 1985. 'Prepuce sucking and tongue rolling in intensively fattened bulls.' *Deutsche Tierarztliche Wockenschrift*, 92, 465–468.

Sharman, D. F., and Stephens, D. B. 1974. 'The effect of apomorphine on the behaviour of farm animals.' *Journal of Physiology*, 242, 25P.

Stephens, D. B. 1974. 'Studies on the effect of social environment on the behavioural growth of artificially-reared British Friesian male calves.' *Animal Production*, 18, 23–34.

Webster, A. J. F. 1987. *Understanding the Dairy Cow*, pp. 330–332. BSP Professional Books, Oxford.

Webster, A. J. F., Saville, C., and Welchman, D. 1986. *Improved Husbandry Systems for Veal Calves*. Farm Animal Care Trust, London.

Wiepkema, P. R., Broom, D. M., Duncan, I. J. H., and van Putten, G. 1983. *Abnormal Behaviours in Farm Animals*. Report of the CEC, Brussels.

GLOSSARY

Agonistic behaviour
The complex of behaviours performed during animal encounters with malevolent intent, including aggression, threat, appeasement, avoidance and display

Allelomimicry
Mutual stimulation and synchronisation of behaviour, copying, e.g. yawning in humans, grazing in cattle

Allogrooming
Licking the trunk of other cattle

Anoestrous
The absence of oestrus, or sexual receptivity, in the female

Binocular vision
See stereoscopic vision

Bos indicus *cattle*
Humped cattle that evolved in India, otherwise known as zebu cattle

Bos taurus *cattle*
European cattle without hump

Conspecifics
Animals of the same species

Electroencephalography
The detection of electrical activity in the brain that arises from mental activity

Elimination
Voiding of excreta

Euphagia
Hunger for a specific nutrient

Flehman
Facial expression where the lips are retracted with the mouth half open and the neck extended to facilitate the passage of odours (especially pheromones) to the vomeronasal or Jacobson's organ via two ducts in the roof of the mouth. Otherwise known as lip curl

Flight distance
Distance from an animal to the edge of its personal space, which when entered causes the animal to flee

Fovea
A concentration of photoreceptive cone cells in the centre of the retina

Genotype
The genetic constitution of an animal

Habituation
Learning not to respond to innate stimuli that have become without function

Hedyphagia
Selection of dietary constituents that have pleasant (hedonistic) characteristics

Heritability
The amount of a trait of the parents (relative to their contemporaries) which on average is passed to the offspring

Ingestion, ingestive behaviour
Feeding; consumption of food

Interaural distance
Distance between the ears

Kinetic activity
Behaviour concerned with movement of the animal

Lower critical temperature
Temperature below which the animal begins to generate additional heat to maintain its core temperature

Macrosmatic
Possessing well-developed olfactory perceptive powers

Microsmatic
Possessing limited olfactory perceptive powers

Multiparous cows
Cows that have given birth more than once

Nociception
Perception of pain

Oestrus
The behavioural manifestation of sexual receptivity and impending ovulation in the cow; also referred to as bulling and heat

Ontogeny
Evolution and development of a characteristic, behaviour or individual

Operant conditioning
Trial and error learning, where repeated presentation of a reinforcing stimulus strengthens a response, e.g. when cattle touch an electric fence, the shock teaches them to avoid the wire in future

Optometric measurements
Determination of the refractive power and visual range of the eye

Osmotic pressure
The pressure required to stop ions diffusing from a solution

Personal space
Volume around an animal which, when entered by another animal, causes the animal to flee

Pheromone
Chemical messenger between animals that often conveys information on sexual receptivity

Photic stimulus
Light stimulus

Photoperiod
Length of the light period during each day; daylight length

Phenotype
The sum of characteristics manifested by an organism that arise from genetic and environmental influences

Photosensitivity
Receptivity to photic stimuli

Prehend (of plants)
   To take into the mouth

Primiparous cow
   Cow that has only given birth once

Reductionist research
   Researching problems in ever greater detail

Rigid back response or stance
   See standing reflex

Social facilitation
   Behaviour that is encouraged by others performing it

Standing reflex
   Acceptance of being mounted by another cow without resistance

Stereoscopic vision
   Combining the sight of two eyes to provide an impression of
   depth and solidarity; binocular vision

Stereotyped behaviour, stereotypies
   Repeated sequences of an activity, often with no direct purpose
   and at unusually high frequency

Ungulate
   Hoofed mammal

Vocalisation
   Calling or making a noise with the voice

Vomeronasal organ
   Olfactory receptive organ situated behind the vomer bone of the
   nose; also known as Jacobson's organ

INDEX

FARMING PRESS BOOKS

Below is a sample of the wide range of agricultural and veterinary books published by Farming Press. For more information or for a free illustrated book list please contact:

Farming Press Books, Wharfedale Road, Ipswich IP1 4LG, United Kingdom   Telephone (0473) 241122   Fax (0473) 240501

Improved Grassland Management   *JOHN FRAME*
Draws on the full range of contemporary research to give practical recommendations.

The Principles of Dairy Farming   *KEN SLATER*
An introduction, setting the husbandry and management techniques of dairy farming in its industry context.

Cattle Feeding   *JOHN OWEN*
A detailed account of the principles and practices of cattle feeding, including optimal diet formulation.

Forage Conservation and Feeding   *RAYMOND, REDMAN, WALTHAM*
Silage- and hay-making, mowing and field treatments, grass drying and forage feeding.

The Herdsman's Book   *MALCOLM STANSFIELD*
The stockperson's guide to the dairy enterprise.

Profitable Beef Production   *M McG COOPER & M B WILLIS*
Analyses and describes the factors making for success in the beef enterprise.

A Veterinary Book for Dairy Farmers   *ROGER BLOWEY*
Deals with the full range of cattle and calf ailments, with the emphasis on preventive medicine.

Cattle Ailments   *EDDIE STRAITON*
The recognition and treatment of all the common cattle ailments shown in over 300 photographs.

Calving the Cow and Care of the Calf   *EDDIE STRAITON*
A highly illustrated manual offering practical, common sense guidance.

Footcare in Cattle: Hoof Structure and Trimming *(VHS VIDEO)*
Roger Blowey first analyses hoof structure and horn growth using laboratory specimens, then demonstrates trimming.

Cattle Footcare and Claw Trimming   *E TOUSSAINT RAVEN*
Combines a guide to the causes, progress, treatment and prevention of foot ailments with practical details on claw trimming.

Calf Rearing   *THICKETT, MITCHELL, HALLOWS*
Covers the housed rearing of calves to twelve weeks, reflecting modern experience in a wide variety of situations.

Farming Press Books is part of the Morgan-Grampian Farming Press Group which publishes a range of farming magazines: Arable Farming, Dairy Farmer, Farming News, Pig Farming, What's New in Farming. For a specimen copy of any of these please contact the address above.